ENERGY MEDICINE FOR YOUR DOG

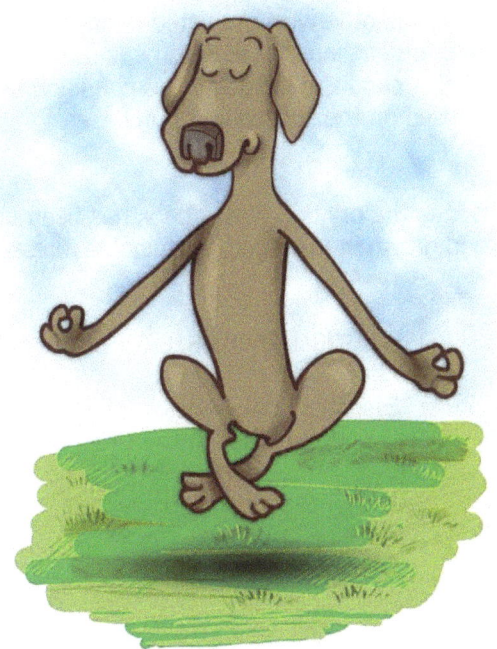

Madison King

A natural, fun way to care for your dog
that both of you will enjoy.

© Madison King 2014

All rights reserved

No part of this publication may be reproduced, stored in a retrieval system, or transmitted in any form or by any means, without the prior permission in writing of the publisher, nor be otherwise circulated in any form of binding or cover other than that in which it is published and without a similar condition including this condition being imposed on the subsequent purchaser.

All paper used in the printing of this book has been made from wood grown in managed, sustainable forests.

ISBN: 978-1-78003-818-6

Essential Book Series
Printed and published in the UK

Author Essentials Ltd
4 The Courtyard
South Street
Falmer
BN1 9PQ

A catalogue record of this book is available from the British Library

Cover design © Author Essentials
info@authoressentials.com

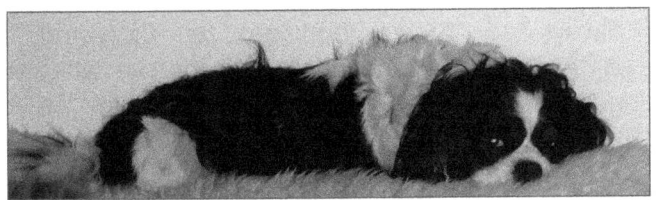

Magnus

In July 1998 I ran my first 'doggie workshop' by the river in Fulham (West London) and over the intervening years have loved working with my own dogs and cats and helping others work with theirs. They are wise souls and while endearingly mischievous at times, irritatingly stubborn at others, most have a purity of energy that is an honour and joy to be with.

I have witnessed energy medicine truly 'rescue' my dog from death (more about that later) and found it has helped everything from an itchy skin condition to testing food, healing cuts, post operative care... and many other everyday aches and pains.

Above all, working with your dog's energies deepens the bond and enhances the communication between you.

In this little book I want to share with you some simple but effective tools to help care for your dog. They are easy, non-intrusive, free and absolutely safe, so do them with love and have fun with them – I'm pretty sure your dog will enjoy every second as indeed you will.

While I use a fun, cartoon theme, don't be deceived, some of these techniques have roots in deeply ancient energy medicine and have been around for years, because they work!

I always say to my humans: *be discerning*. Try everything in this little book and observe what your dog seems to enjoy the most – let her[1] (him) be your guide.

It is an interesting phenomenon that very often your dog will 'reflect' what is wrong with <u>you</u>.

- *Is there a hidden message about <u>you</u>, something <u>you</u> need to address?*
- *Maybe it is <u>you</u> who needs the energy medicine?*
- *Is your mutt being a mirror?*
- *Is he picking up your depression?*
- *Is his stiff hip mimicking yours?*
- *Is his itchy skin secretly telling you that you have a problem with 'letting go'?*
- *Is his constipation doing the same?*

Think about it, I always do and invariably I am surprised and rewarded by some 'ahh haa' moments with regard to my own health.

Animals have always been part of my life: from my first bunny Winston, ponies, horses, and various cats and dogs have shared my happiness and been there as a comfort in my sadness. I have been through the heart-wrenching grief of losing them and the radiant joy of meeting them for the first time. They show me what true love is and the meaning of a soul mate;

---

[1] Simply for ease of reading, I will refer to 'her' throughout the book.

they have healed my soul on many occasions and their antics and expressions have made me laugh with childish joy.

We all have this special bond with our beloved pets and it is this loving link that can make 'healing' them so easy. You don't really have to think about it too much; the energy of that love does half the work for you! None of what you are about to read is difficult, some things you will do already without 'labelling'. Feel safe that nothing on these pages will harm your companion. The work will help and enhance the bond between you and improve health, happiness and general well being for you both. Most of all, relax and have fun and your dog will too.

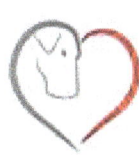

I should say that the information in this book is not intended to replace the visits to your vet, rather to give you some everyday 'tools' to help keep your dog healthy and if she does have to go to the vet, to support the treatment.

We will cover the following basics:

Brief background and factoids

HANDS ON CANINE COMFORTING
- A spinal flush
- Give your dog a massage
- The basic massage formula
- Tibetan Figure 8's
- Hopi Indian Technique
- 8 the eyes
- Hook her up
- Give her some verbal
- Getting to the point

Energy Medicine For Your Dog

HANDS OFF!
- Working with the chakras
- Aura sensing
- Calm the Canine Conan within
- 3 point magic
- How to lick your dog

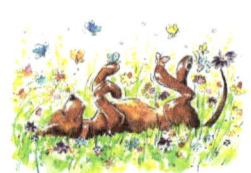

ASSORTED DOGGIE BITS 'N PIECES
- Doggie Elementals – your dog and the 5 Elements.
- Tracing some very strange flows
- Working with the pathways of energy
- How to build her immunity
- The ideal doggie diet
- Surrogate testing
- Using a pendulum
- A canine care kit
- Flower essences
- Essential Oils
- Crystals
- Stress tap for you
- Choosing a vet

Why did I write this book and who am I?

- Walking the tightrope:
- 4 THUMPS
- CROSS CRAWL
- TIBETAN MEDIATION POSE
- HOOK UP

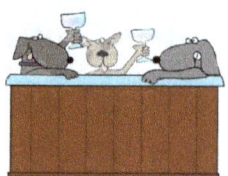

How to do a basic energy test

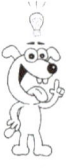

All interspersed with little 'bites' of information designed to give you something to chew on.
(OK, I promise I won't make any more canine quips).

Energy Medicine For Your Dog

I hope you enjoy the following pages and please let me know what you and your pooch think of some of the techniques – I love getting feedback!

Finally, I want to thank the many wonderful teachers, students and clients over the years that have helped me learn and grow in the natural healthcare field. In particular, Donna Eden (founder of Eden Energy Medicine)[2] and of course: Winston, Chloe, Fred, Charley, Harley, Magnus, Tash, Proctor, Boris, Nasher, Morris, Mumkin and Mabel, my little four-legged soulmates.

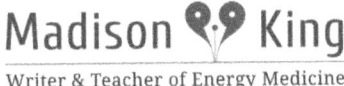

Writer & Teacher of Energy Medicine

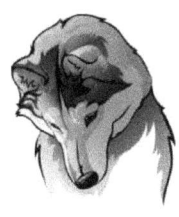

Whether she be a Saint Bernard or a tiny Chihuahua, your dog probably descended from one single animal: THE WOLF. The different breeds in existence today are 'manmade'.

* The first dogs on record were Mesopotamian greyhounds about 8,000 years ago.

* The earliest *images* of dogs are in a Spanish cave and thought to date back 12,000 years.

* In 4500BC the Egyptians worshipped Anubis, who was represented as a greyhound with erect ears

---

[2] www.innersource.net

Energy Medicine For Your Dog

and a forked tail. (Very much like today's Spanish Pharaoh Hound) They gave immense respect to their dogs and when one died, the owners shaved off their eyebrows, covered their head in mud and mourned. I have to say, I've felt like that on occasions.

* The Chinese nobility bred small dogs as pets and guardians, hence the twin Fu lion-dog statues that guard doorways 'in the know'. Their dogs had their own servants. Well, that's nothing new, Mabel has me!

* The Dali Llama was guarded in his palace at Lhasa by Lhasa Apsos. One might think of them as spiritual Rottweilers.

* In Native American Indian culture, the dog totem symbolises SERVICE and LOYALTY. Those born under the sign of the dog in Chinese astrology are thought to be loyal. Loyalty and dogs go hand in hand.

* Alexander the Great used dogs from India in battle. It is said that he founded and named a city Peritas, in memory of his dog.

* Great Danes and Mastiffs wore spiked armour in the Middle Ages and entered battle with their owners.

* In Greece, dogs were used as watch dogs; Homer, Aesop and Aristotle all wrote about dogs. Plato once said: "*a dog has the soul of a philosopher*". The ancient Greek phrase: *'dog days of Summer'* described the hottest days that fell in alignment with the rising of the Dog Star – Sirius.

- *Cave Canem* (beware of the dog) signs have been found in Pompeii! The Romans were believed to have kept dogs purely for companionship.

- It's raining cats and dogs – this originated in the 17th century in England when, during heavy rain and flooding, many homeless animals drowned and the streets would be littered by them.

Now, in most parts of the Western world, dogs work with us: guiding, hearing, hunting, retrieving, sniffing. There are PAT, sheep, police, guard dogs and they also share our lives as treasured companions.

"Until one has loved an animal, a part of one's soul remains unawakened."

Anatole France

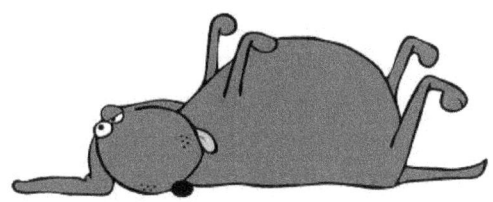

HANDS ON
CANINE COMFORTING

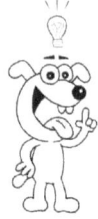

Touch is the first sense a dog develops. Her entire body is covered with touch sensitive nerve endings; she will truly feel your 'hands on' work with her.

For all the techniques I share with you here, I would add one proviso and that is: **if your dog walks away and doesn't want anything to do with it – respect that**.

Perhaps just starting with simple stroking, to get her used to your hands with a different intention behind them, is a good idea.

Your safety net is that she will always know when she has had enough and have no qualms about getting up and leaving. Or the eyes to the ceiling cringing might give you a hint.

Marvel at the wisdom and don't suffer hurt feelings or deflated ego. As with so much in life, the wisdom is knowing when to let go.

Spending quality 'touch time' with your dog is essential for both of you... it calms and relaxes you both, not just your dog will benefit.

You can always find time: do it while you watch your favourite television programme.

You may like to start with a couple of minutes of grooming with the brush of your choice

Sit, Stand Lie Down – which is best? It is entirely up to you and the size of your dog. As a rule of thumb, small dogs are good sitting on your lap or sofa next to you, whereas a larger dog is often more accessible standing up with hips between your legs. Small or large dog, both, once they relax, will probably want to lie down.

If a dog is a little suspicious of what you are doing, do it with her standing up rather than sitting or lying down; she will feel less vulnerable standing. As she gets accustomed to your special 'energy medicine touch', she will relax and sit/lie down voluntarily.

As an introductory massage, gently massage his head with small circular motions and work your way over his entire body. Roam wherever you feel inclined. Keep it short – about a minute. This is not a remedial treatment so be gentle.

You can use your fingertips or entire palm, depending upon the size of your dog and what 'feels' good to you (and her). On some of the larger muscle groups such as shoulder and hip, the heel of your hand gives a good firm touch.

Whatever of the treatments you actually use with your dog – try closing your eyes when you are touching her. By removing the sense of sight, your other senses become more 'sensitive'. In this way you will 'tune in' to her feelings and needs more easily.

Done regularly, you get to know your dog's body and therefore will notice anything irregular very quickly and can act on it.

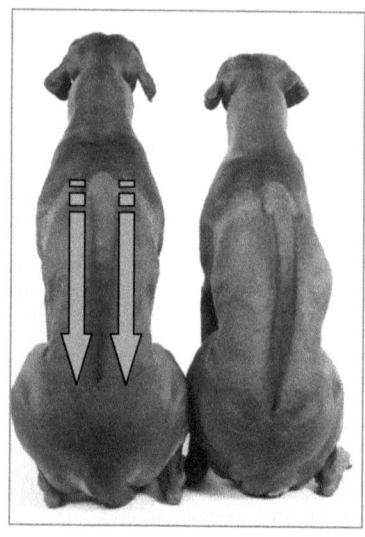

A SPINAL FLUSH

I'm putting this in pole position because all my dogs have loved the technique; it has been 'numero uno' in my house for many years. It can be done anytime, anywhere and for just a few seconds or a few minutes.

Standing or sitting, the choice is yours. It's always a winner.

* Start licking your dog (not literally, see the section below) and, with relaxed fingers, stroke over the top of the head and down the back to the base of the spine and then brush off the entire length of the tail. Do it simultaneously on both sides of the head and spine. Repeat several times, increasing the pressure gently with each stroke.

* Repeat a few times to get her relaxed and used to your touch, she will know you have a different 'intention'.

* Stroke up between the eyes to the top of the head (over her 3rd eye, located between the 'eyebrows') repeat 3 times. You can use thumbs or fingers – whatever feels comfortable. (This sends Mabel into a semi-zombie like state in a nano second).

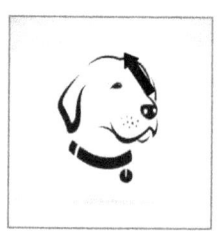

Energy Medicine For Your Dog

- I always talk to her at the same time. It really doesn't matter what words you use, we all know it's the tone of voice that is important.

- You can use two hands or one, it really depends upon the size of your dog but with fingertips gently rub down on either side of the spine. You will be stimulating key lymphatic reflexes that are linked to different organs of the body, bringing balance and calm. Plus stimulating blood flow, helping to remove toxins and relieving any residue muscle tightness.

- Rub over one set of points for a few seconds and then move down an inch to the next pair.

- You can rub up and down or in a circular motion, both are valid, see which one feels best for you and of course which variation gets the best canine response.

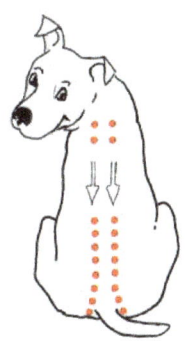

- Pressure is firm but not enough to cause pain and don't rub on the bone itself; you are working in the 'gully' on either side of the spine itself.

- Start at the neck and work all the way down the spine and brush off the tail.

- End by stroking from head to tail tip a couple of times.

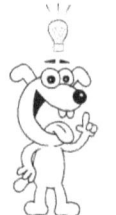

Dogs have an active 6th sense. They are capable of finding their way home over vast distances. We have all heard 'fantastic' tales of animals 'coming home'. There is no rational or linear explanation, although we do know they have the ability to detect subtle changes in the earth's magnetic field. I think it is because their 3rd eye is open, they can tune in and allow it to guide them. Dogs are spiritual beings, so anything is possible!

"There is no psychiatrist in the world like a puppy licking your face"

Ben Williams

You might like to explore Tellington Touch – I am a huge fan of this touch technique. www.ttouch.com Linda Tellington originally developed and used it with horses but it works a treat on dogs (and other 4-leggeds too)... She has videos up on You Tube just tap in Tellington TTouch.

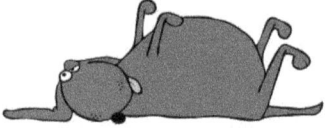

GIVE YOUR DOG A MASSAGE.

The ideal time to work on your dog is after an energetic walk, when she is ready to relax and not bouncing around with pent up energy – common sense really, unless you feel like making life difficult for yourself.

Sit quietly together and say her name softly.[3] Talk to her in your mind, visualising pictures that bring your words to life. Dogs understand visual communication with great ease. It's us humans that need to perfect the art. With practice you will find you communicate with your dog and her thoughts/pictures will begin to spring into your mind. Don't doubt, question or invalidate this when it happens, don't let the left brain and your intellect deny this form of communication – it does happen, just open your heart to 'receive' and let go of any preconceived ideas or expectations.

There are various ways you may 'receive' from your pet:

- You may *hear* her words in your head
- You may *see* pictures
- You may *feel* her feelings
- You may just have a *'knowing'*

Of course TOUCH is a universal inter-species communication and your massage will say so much. It is essential to the bond between you.

Centre yourself and bring a loving intention to the field around you both. You will be working for a few minutes, your dog will let you know when she has had enough – never force it. Over time she will want longer sessions. Mabel now comes and sits in front of me and places her paw on my wrist when she wants a massage.

---

[3] I remember many years ago training Harley by the river in Fulham and a man in a wheelchair was watching me. He had a dog trained to help him and he gave me a very good tip: *Don't rely on shouting your commands. Make the dog 'stretch' to hear you, call her name in a whisper, issue the command in a whisper. Firmly but quietly.* **Decrease the volume and your dog's attention will increase.**

- A daily massage gives you an opportunity to really know her body and will alert you to anything unusual such as lumps, lesions, dry patches and even little unwelcome 'visitors' that may appear.

- You will increase the blood circulation which benefits the entire body and promotes a healthy coat.

- By stimulating lymphatic flow and encouraging the efficient removal of toxins, you will be helping her immune system.

- You will obviously be relaxing tense muscles and creating space in the limbs for energy to move and aid flexibility.

- You will be reducing anxiety and releasing stress. If you subscribe to the notion that most of what goes wrong with an animal is caused, or exacerbated, by stress, then decreasing her stress reaction you can help anything.

- An enjoyable way to enhance your bond with her.

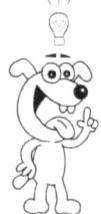

A dog will repeat whatever gets attention. So make sure you only give her attention when she does something good.

THE BASIC MASSAGE FORMULA

Sitting or standing, get as comfortable and relaxed as possible.

Do a few preliminary strokes from head to tip of tail with the palm of your hands, each stroke a little firmer.

Rest your hands on her neck and pelvis for a few moments.

Start with an initial hold:

> *One hand on her chest*
> *One hand on the back of*
> *her head/neck area*

* Synchronise your breathing with hers.

* Gently stroke or circle over these two areas.

* Keeping one hand on her chest, use the other to stroke her lightly all over:

  * *Head to tip of tail*
  * *Head neck shoulders down each front leg and off the paws*
  * *Head spine hips back legs and off the paws*
  * *Head to tip of tail again*

* Massage in small, firm circles around and over the surface of the ears, both inside and outside – this can be very calming as the ears are brimming with acupuncture points relating to the entire body; by massaging them you are effectively giving her a treatment throughout her entire body.

- You could incorporate a spinal flush at this point

- Work gently around the hips and shoulders and between the 'toes'. When you massage a human your hand glides over the skin. It is a different technique when you are working with fur. Yes, you can stroke over the hair but if you want to go deeper you place your hand, palm, fingertips (whatever you decide to use) firmly on the fur and move it over the underlying tissue. This is bliss around the big muscle groups on the thighs.

- On the subject of hips and shoulders: place the palm of your hand over the area and slowly slowly apply pressure and then move the skin in a circle. Release the pressure and repeat. No sudden movements and release the pressure immediately if your dog doesn't like it. If your dog has been running and very active, this is heaven for her.

- Another good technique on big joint areas is to put your fingers into a 'claw', firmly grasp/connect with the joint and move in circular movements, or however you feel drawn. Do it on yourself and see how good it feels.

- If she has lower leg problems, wrap your fingers around the top of the leg and squeeze, very gently, the muscles; release, move down an inch and repeat until you get to the paw and then 'brush off' the entire leg.

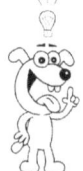

Dogs carry 75% of their weight on the shoulder joints at the front of the body and those joints respond positively to massage.

Energy Medicine For Your Dog

- Get her to lie on her back and stroke very gently over the abdominal area with small gentle circles and figure 8s, both large and small; I don't need to remind you that this is a submissive pose for a dog, a very vulnerable one in their minds, so no sudden or hard movements to break her trust.

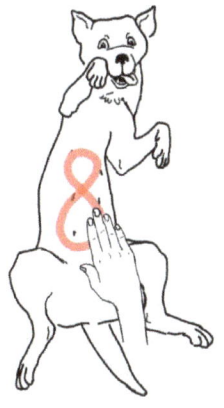

- With her lower spine resting on your open palms, rock her side to side, slowly and rhythmically in this position. It can be profoundly relaxing to a dog if she feels safe with you; and may help any hip or spine stiffness, although obviously check with your vet if your dog suffers severe problems in this area.

- Hold the back of the head with one hand and the base of the tail/lower back with the other, tune into her breathing and feel the energy running between your hands. You might even find yourself drawn to mentally tracing Figure 8's either horizontally or vertically along the spine. Large or small, let your intuition guide you. There is no right or wrong.

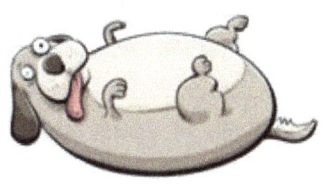

Energy Medicine For Your Dog

OK, THAT'S THE' BASIC RECIPE' – HERE ARE A FEW THINGS YOU CAN ADD:

You have already tried the figure 8 – why do I like it so much?

The Tibetans had a firm belief in the power of the symbol '8' – it is infinity – energy often moves in an 8 and 8s have the added benefit of stimulating the 'Strangeflows'[4] that are the energies of joy and repair, the true trouble-shooters in the body. If your dog has an injury of any kind, figure 8 over it for as long as is comfortable and it really helps heal the injury or wound. You will need to do it frequently (at first every couple of hours, then 2 or 3 times a day) but it is worth the effort.

It works for humans too. I once gave a workshop and mentioned about how effective Figure 8'ing was over wounds. One of the students had a friend who had a major wound on her torso which would not heal; the doctors were beginning to get concerned. She figure 8'd it every evening when she was watching the news and within a week it had started to draw together and heal.

- ❈ Start by tracing (with your hand, focus and intention) 8s up and down the spine. On or off the skin, doesn't matter.

- ❈ You can trace them anywhere you suspect a problem. Particularly useful over wounds and sore joints and limbs.

---

[4] These are ancient flows of energy identified by Traditional Chinese Medicine and go by many different names: Extraordinary Vessels, Psychic Conduits, Radiant circuits to name but a few. There are 4 main flows and 4 'hybrid' flows.

Energy Medicine For Your Dog

* They can be tiny little ones over small areas or larger ones encompassing her entire body; and can be traced in any direction.

THE HOPI INDIAN TECHNIQUE

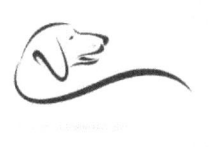

The Hopi Indians in New Mexico are renowned for their healing tradition; the word 'Hopi' means 'peaceful ones'.

They developed this simple yet profoundly effective technique. It is a 'wisdom' that has been handed down through oral tradition by the Hopi Elders.

It connects directly with the brain, encouraging it to release muscle spasm and tightness in the back and relieve pain. In releasing the spine, one is affecting the entire body. Therefore, if pain is present throughout large areas of the body, this technique can provide a measure of relief.

It adapts beautifully to canine use.

* Dog sitting or lying down

* Ground yourself (if you are not sure how, email me and I will send you some techniques for grounding: madisonking@hotmail.com)

* Rub your hands together and shake them off. This removes any stale, tired energies and leaves your hands fresh and renewed.

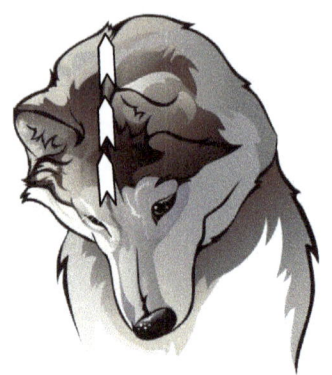

- Do a Doggie Crown Pull by working gently along the 'Mohican' centre line of her head. From forehead to where her collar sits.

- This opens up the head and allows the energy you will be stimulating, with the Hopi technique, to move out.

- Put your fingertips on either side of the central line and pull apart, outwards towards the side of her head. Move up an inch and repeat until you have moved over the entire 'line' until you reach her neck. Pressure is 'firmly gentle'.

- Place the palm of your hand at the base of her neck, about 2" off the skin itself. Just leave your hand there, tune in and connect with your dog and then very very slowly move down over the spine, keeping off the skin. What can you feel? Heat, cold, tingling or nothing? – doesn't matter. You are beginning to move the energy down the spine.

- Place the tips of your fingers, in line with the spine and on either side of the spine. Your fingers are pointing downward into the body itself. In this way you have made a 'spinal sandwich' with your fingertips. Use both hands so the spine sits neatly in between both sets of fingertips.

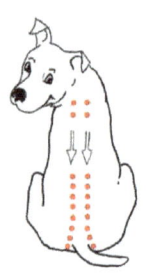

- Bring all your attention and focus to what you are doing, mentally visualise energies beaming down into you from above, along your arms, shooting along each finger and, like laser beams, coming out of your fingertips into the body of your pooch. Healing, strengthening energy, focussed and laser-like. This calls in 'yang' energy which is outgoing and invigorating. You may be drawn to pulling in the quieter, more 'introvert' and calming Yin energy, in which case you visualise the energies coming up from Mother Earth. If you are not clear which one to pull in, try them both and see which one your dog prefers.

- Using a feather light touch, no real pressure at all, in fact you may like to experiment with holding the fingertips ¼" off the fur; inch your hands along the length of the spine to the next section (each section being the width of your 4 fingertips). As you do so, keep your focus, mentally 'laser beam' energy through your fingers into your pooch's back.

- I'm suggesting a light or non-existent touch, however, if you feel like digging in deeper or rocking from side to side – DO IT! Mabel (my dog) loves a firm pressure on two areas: between the shoulder blades and where her tail joins. Be guided by your dog.

- Continue along the spine, taking time on each 'section' to intuit what might be needed.

- The Hopi technique is a playground for your instinct and intuition.

Energy Medicine For Your Dog

- Before finishing, pinch and lift the skin over the spine itself – gently. Begin at the neck and travel down the spine to the base of the tail.

- End by Figure 8'ing the entire spine and let your hands gently come to rest on the body.

- One hand on the sacrum and one at the top of the spine.

- Brush off the back, legs and feet.

- A variation on this is to put both thumbs on the side of the spine closest to you and all your fingers on the opposite side of the spine. Use both hands. Travel the full length in either direction. Then move to the other side of your friend and repeat the process.

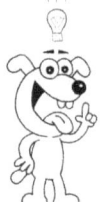

> It is always a good idea, after any 'energy work' to wash your hands under cool water to cleanse them of any tired energy you may have picked up.

An ancient Egyptian sun technique

I have spent a lot of time in Egypt, have even led workshops in Giza and have 'flown the sands' on Arab horses. There is a strong, almost raw, energy in the land and their ancient history is fascinating, they were people who truly understood energy. One technique I think you will enjoy is this...

- Your dog should be standing

- Form an '0' with your index finger and thumb (on both hands). Your little fingers will be touching the skin so the '0' is a few inches off the body.
- Place one '0' over the base of her back, just where the tail emerges.
- Place the other '0' on the back between the shoulder.
- Close your eyes.
- Hold for 30 seconds with focus on bringing in the Yang energy of the sun, down through the '0' and into her body; invigorating and energising your dog.

Now, from ancient Egypt to the USA...

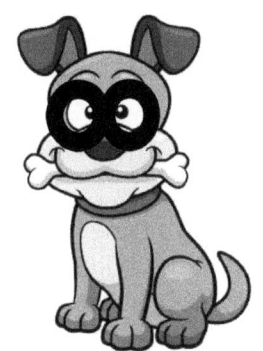

MR MCGOO – 8 THE EYES TO GET THE ENERGIES CROSSING

Continuing on the healing properties of the Tibetan '8': trace a horizontal '8' over your dogs eyes.

Start on the bridge of the nose, up over one eye, down and back to the centre and then on the other side.

Energy Medicine For Your Dog

Work about 2" off the fur and go quite slowly and deliberately.

This gets all the energy moving in the eye area thereby promotes eye health. It also helps the energy start crossing in the entire body, on a cellular level, which in turn helps achieve a healthier energetic balance and also encourages left and right brain integration that all mammals need as a foundation of health.

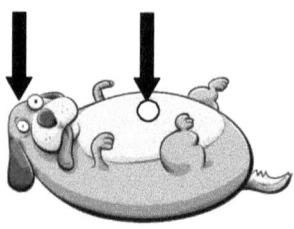

Hook her up

When she is really relaxed and out for the count on her back, gently hold, with open palms, her 3rd eye and navel, connect, close your eyes and hold for as long as she'll let you.

This hooks up two key pathways of energy and activates a radiant, healing energy in her body. It gives courage and helps interaction with you and other animals. Very good for the fearful dog that goes on the offensive to disguise her 'fear'.

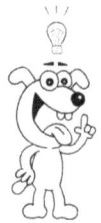

The print of your dog's nose
is as unique as your finger prints.
And that nose can smell 1000 times better
than you!

GIVE HER SOME VERBAL

Whenever you are working with your pet, talk to her:

*May your eyes see only good things.
May your ears hear my loving words.
May you smell your friends and know you are part of a tribe.
May you feel my soothing touch.
May you heal and replenish with ease.
May we live together in peace, happiness and harmony.
May you enjoy our bond as we share this part of life's journey together.
You are not alone dear friend, I am here – you are safe.
I love you.*

GETTING TO THE POINT

Massage briskly and then Figure 8 with your fingertips over these 5 points – 10 seconds on each will bring balance. If you are not sure of the location, sit in front of your dog, hands on either side of the shoulder and start massaging in circles all over the shoulder, down the ribcage and over the hips. Adding a bit of pressure and a figure 8 in the general area of the points.

* **GB34** to relieve pain and tension in *muscles, ligaments and tendons.* Situated on the outside of the back leg near the joint.

* **BL 11** for strong *bones*. On the top of the shoulder. *(both these points are especially good for German Shepherd dogs)*

- **CENTRAL 17** for *lung and heart* – on the chest between the legs

- **CENTRAL 12** for *intestines* – a little bit further back towards the navel

- **LIV 13** for *internal organs* – back towards the hips nearly at the end of the ribcage

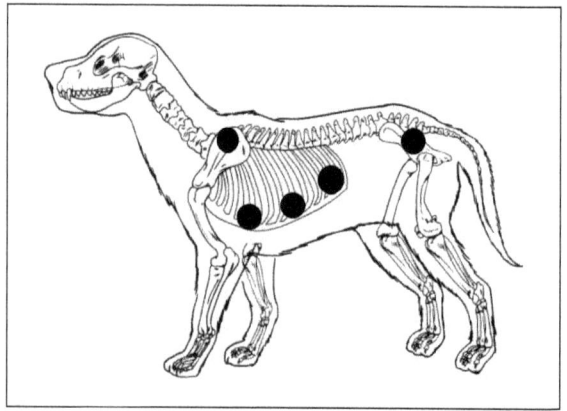

Did you know that dogs have sweat glands, in between their paws

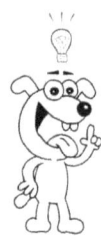

HANDS OFF!

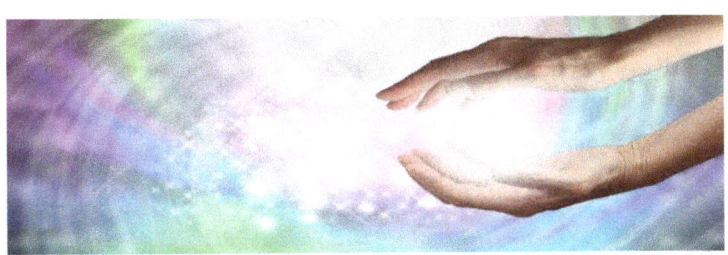

WORKING WITH THE CHAKRAS

Chakra is the Sanskrit word for 'wheel' and that's exactly what Chakras are; spinning wheels of energy located in different parts of the dog's body.

Different parts of the body relate to different chakras. Work on all of them (they work as a team) and add extra focus to any area that you feel needs an extra 'shot' of healing attention.

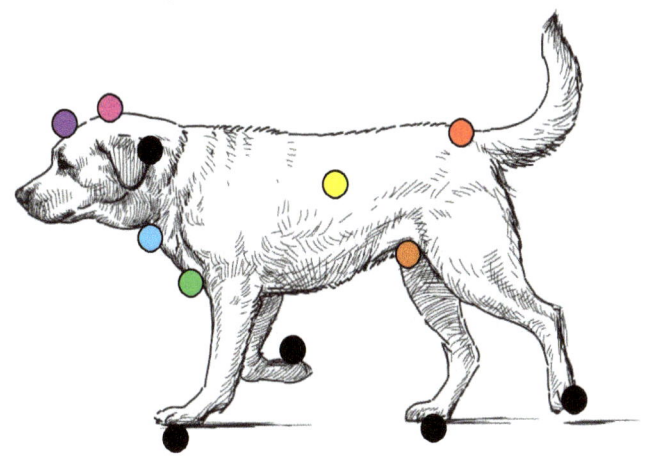

Energy Medicine For Your Dog

- **Root** chakra is located at the base of the tail on the top
- **Sacral** chakra over the womb area
- **Solar plexus** on the 'withers'
- **Heart** over the heart
- **Throat** over the throat
- **Brow** over the brow
- **Crown** on the top of the head between the ears

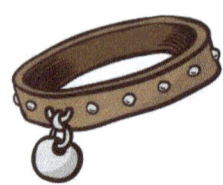

A word about colours – each chakra is individual with many layers and can be any colour, so don't have too many preconceptions.

Colour is powerful – why not test her collar or harness to ensure it is strengthening her not weakening her.

How to do it? Using a surrogate, ensure her throat area is testing strong. Hold different coloured materials over the area and test – which ones strengthen and which weaken?

As a generalisation: **RED or ORANGE** – very energising, not a good idea on an over-active dog. **BLUE or GREEN** – might be better for an over active dog or any dog that needs balance. Good colour for throat problems

The objective of working with the chakra system is to get, and keep, energy moving on these energy stations and avoid tired, stagnant energies accumulating to block the flow of energy and ultimately cause a physical problem for the dog.

Because chakra energy spins out of the body, it is a relatively easy energy to sense and feel with your hands, but how do you know if a chakra is out of balance and needs attention?

There are three ways:

By feel and instinct. When you hold your hand over the chakra, what do you 'feel' about the energy? Is the energy:

- *Strong or weak*
- *Moving or stagnant*
- *Hot or cold*
- *Easy to locate or difficult (collapsed)*

Energy testing using a surrogate Touch the area of the chakra and test.

Using a pendulum – simply hold the pendulum over the chakra (about 6 inches away) Relax and wait.

What happens? If a chakra is strong the energy will be spinning outwards and connect with your pendulum making it spin in a strong circle. If your pendulum does not move or spins in a very sluggish way, they you can suspect a weak and tired chakra.

* Chakras are very effective to work with when you are dealing with damaged emotions, so always check them if your dog is a rescue, has had a traumatic past or has recently been upset.

* If you are particularly well tuned to your pooch you may be able to sink down into the layers of specific chakras, where her past is stored, and sense key issues that have affected her.

* In general, animals have larger and more vibrant chakras in relationship to their body size than us humans and therefore respond very quickly to this type of work.

* Working with them encourages the body's energies to balance; strengthening your pet's inner resources and abilities to repair, heal and replenish – from within, organically and naturally.

* Simply the act of putting your hands on your pet, with a loving intention can transfer energy into her body and stimulate this much desired balance.

Okay, I can sense you might be keen to know *how* to work with these sensitive centres.

Relax your dog, perhaps with a short spinal flush, or simply stroking her and get yourself grounded too. This is not something to do before a walk when she is bouncing around in anticipation of a good run.

I call this 'Stirring the Soup' and while one of the simplest of techniques, it can have profound benefits, particularly in the emotional arena, for your dog.

- Hold the left hand over the chakra area and circle ANTI clockwise for a minute
- Hold the right hand over the chakra and circle clockwise for 30 seconds
- Weave small figure 8's over the chakra for 15 seconds
- Either hand – hold quietly over the area for a further 15–30 seconds, sending love and healing into the energy vortex.

The usual sequence is shown below, but as always, if you feel drawn to do the 'sacred triad' of Root, Sacral and Solar Plexus first and then the others. Follow that instinct. It is not so 'tidy' as the human system.

The Sacred Triad is located at the ROOT of the tail + on the 'withers' and over the womb (sacral).

1 – ROOT	These two work as a combination on dogs. Associated with survival instincts and sexual issues.
2 – SACRAL	
Also known as Womb Chakra	Without doubt work this area on rescue dogs. Very grounding, when they lie down they will be drawing Earth energy up through their Sacral chakra as well as through the minor chakras in their paws. Earth energy in yin in nature, so cooling, calming and 'contracting', coming back into their space, back into a tribe.

	Important for their physical energy and 'presence'. Right at the base of the spine, dogs interact and communicate from the Root (you will know what I mean if you are a dog owner ... *sniff sniff*). The Root Chakra is stimulated when they roll and rub on the ground. The scent around this area and the 'bottom' is like a canine 'calling card', a vital clue to identity.
3 – SOLAR PLEXUS	This is fear and ego and the one to work if you have a fearful or excessively dominant dog. Entry point for Yang energy into the body. If this is constantly out of balance, make sure you clear the minor chakras on the paws so that she can take in balancing Yin energies.
4 – HEART	It is said that this is NOT a major chakra on dogs as they are so evolved – they ARE all heart. However, I personally feel that connecting into this chakra, gently enhances the loving bond between the two of you. Work this chakra if you are weaning puppies, if there is a new pet coming in, if one has been lost and you might like to include flower essences (see later in the book). Take a minute to connect your heart energy to hers.

5 – THROAT	Dogs communicate telepathically so this is not such an important chakra as it is on humans. Nevertheless it can get blocked and cause a problem over the area.
6 – 3RD EYE/ BROW **7 – CROWN**	These two work so closely together with dogs as they operate on psychic levels and are totally 'connected' to the 'Universe'. Their connection with you too. Deeply stressed dogs will sometimes shut down in these chakras – notice the dull emptiness in the eyes of deeply traumatised dogs. Some dogs are uncomfortable with this area being touched, so go gently. There is an inherent balance that Nature keeps here and we humans need to be sensitive to that delicate dance of energies.
Minor chakras	These are located on the paws (which link to the Root chakra on the belly). They are the main entry points for YIN energy into the dog. The tip of the tail Paw chakras sense the earth energy and will lead a dog to a 'good' energy spot, where it will then lie down so that it's Root/sacral chakras can better absorb that energy. There are little bud chakras at the inside base of each ear

Energy Medicine For Your Dog

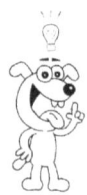

How about buying (or making) a rainbow coloured blanket for your dog to sleep on, or put down different coloured towels/throws and see if there is one she favours – it could be she needs the vibrational healing quality of that particular colour.

Just as we humans have many minor chakras, so do dogs. Perhaps the most useful for us to massage are the paws, all four of them. Vital for drawing up cooling and calming Yin Earth energy and feeding the entire system.

Also, at the end of the tip of the tail, it acts as an antennae pulling in the more expansive yang energy from the 'sun'.

So you dog is pulling in 'yang' energy from the sun in through her tail and 'yin' energy from the moon up through her paws. So while these are classified as 'minor' don't disregard them as a healthy dog has a good balance between her yang and yin energies.

On the subject of yin and yang, your fingers have different 'charges'.

- *Index finger is yang*
- *Middle finger is yin*
- *Ring finger is yang*
- *Little finger is yin*
- *Using a triad of Index, middle and ring creates a 'neutral' hold*

Experiment when you are working on your dog – most of the time you are working with all your fingertips but when you are working with one or two, observe her reaction to the Index finger as opposed to the Middle finger working an area. They bring different qualities and she will sense that.

The chakra energy in a human is very simple – think of a column of energy running up the middle of the body. However, in your dog, the chakras are not quite so distinctly placed and they do hold a different hierarchy.

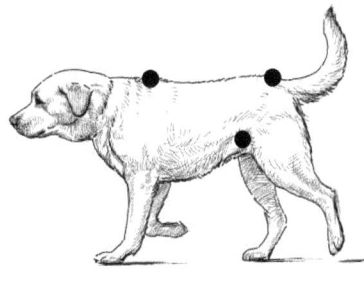

Think of a triangle, a 'sacred triad' formed by the 3 major chakras: **Root, Sacral (womb) and Solar plexus**.

A start point for your session would be to ensure these 3 are all in balance.

The Minor chakras of paws and tail are next – as explained above, entry points for energy both Yin and Yang. Paw balance essential for an animal to feel safe and rooted.

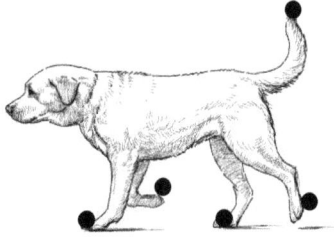

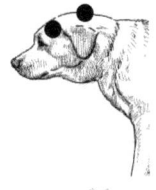

The remaining Crown and Brow chakras next and end with the throat and ear bud chakras.

To summarise; the treatment is the same 5 steps for them all:
1. Connect
2. Left hand ANTI clockwise
3. Right hand clockwise
4. Fig 8
5. Hold and sense

Another technique is to hold any two chakras at the same time, breathe and connect their energies with your intention flowing through your hands.

Don't forget to *always* re-test after you have made a correction, so you know it has worked and your dog is strengthened by the work you have done together.

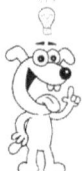

> Did you know that a dog could interpret your smile as an aggressive baring of your teeth. Mind you I did it to Mabel and she just sighed, turned her back and conveyed the sense of 'yeah, whatever!'.

HEART TO HEART[5]

Sit in front of your dog with her sitting up looking at you so her chest is facing you. Imagine a figure of 8 joining her heart to yours. It can be made of anything you like, any colour, any texture but link your heart to her heart. Repeating the word LOVE, or whatever you feel appropriate: cherish, nurture, safety, healing, strength, joy etc., whatever you feel might be comforting to her.

This is a warm true bonding between the two of you.

---

[5] One of my favourite heart designs is this one – it is the logo for a great jewellery designer – www.Kleshna.com

Energy Medicine For Your Dog

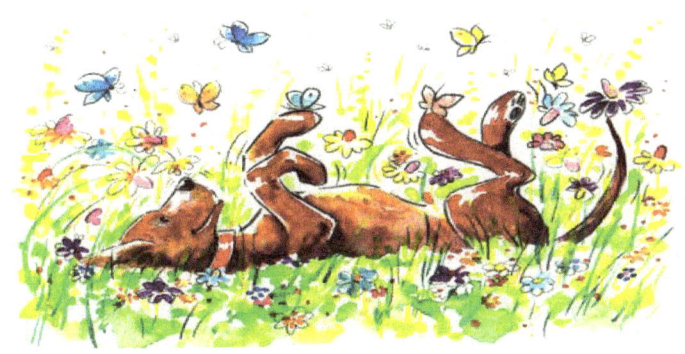

AURA SENSING

One of the easiest ways of working with your dog is simple 'hands on' aura sensing; done from the heart with lashings of love. If you are unfamiliar with this, there is no mystery; here's an easy way to start:

Sit quietly with your dog and say a small 'prayer' to ensure that the healing you give will come only from the highest source of love.

You could say something like:

May I bring healing energies of the highest love and light to Mabel today, in the most divine way.

Lay your hands gently on your dog, anywhere that draws you, or you know there is a problem, and take a couple of deep breaths. Then lift your hands off the actual fur and skin and hover over the body about an inch or two away.

You are connecting to her aura: Slowly run your hand 2" – 3" above her body from head to tail, sensing where there is any change of energy in your hands – e.g. hot cold, something pushing/pulling, sluggishness, change of taste in your mouth, unexpected emotions you may feel.

You may sense nothing the first few times you do this, *it doesn't matter* – one day you will and it's worth persevering, it's a wonderful feeling when you first feel her energy; and once you have, there is no going back, your ability grows. Until then, just *trust* that running your hands over her in this manner will be balancing in some way and a possible catalyst to repair.

When you detect a change, keep your hand over that place until you feel it shift for the positive and then move on. You may feel inclined to trace a small figure 8 or circle your hand, give your intuition free rein. Don't judge it, force it or doubt it.

If there is pain in an area, 'unwind' the pain out of the body:

* With your left hand over the painful area, make anti clockwise circles, connecting to the dog's energy and slowly spiral it out of the animal, moving your hand further and further away and then shaking the pain off your hand. The energy of pain can sometimes form a 'vortex' over the area and this spirally of your hand begins to clear it.

* Now place the right hand over the area and circle clockwise over the area – just a dozen times, which will have the effect of stabilising the shift you have just made.

Rescan the area and it should feel constant.

Use your instinct on how to end any 'session'. I often gently stroke around the ears, cradle her face and kiss her forehead (but that's me, I'm soft!). As with all work of this kind, thank the 'Universal Energy' for any healing that has taken place.

Sometimes that healing is not immediately evident – there are no trumpet fanfares or instant miracles but there may be a subtle shift that will result in an improvement in a day or two, or even longer. You may have been a catalyst to resetting her inner healer.

A 'healing' method that is superb if your dog doesn't want to be touched or is away from you, in the veterinary surgery or hospital, is to imagine her the size of a chess piece sitting in your cupped hands in front of your chest. This is effectively your Heart centre. With your imaginary pet in your hands, send pure love, healing, replenishing energy to that little effigy, perhaps figure 8'ing between your heart and the figure, to deepen the connection. Smile as you do it and don't doubt the bond of love and its power to support her natural healing abilities.

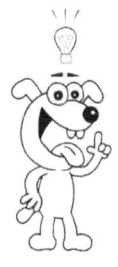

Always visualise your dog as fit, well and healthy. Manifestation follows thought, so if your dog has a swelling, visualise the swelling subsiding. If he has stiff joints visualise them mobile and flexible.

CALM THE CANINE CONAN WITHIN

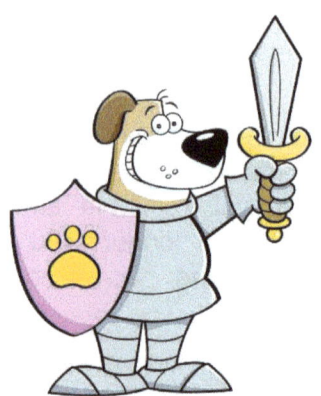

When your dog is stressed, the pathway of energy called Triple Warmer goes into overdrive.

To fuel that overdrive it takes energy from other pathways and their associated organs and systems; thus weakening the entire body.

The first one it drains is Spleen meridian, which instantly reduces your dog's ability to process the stress – so she gets stuck in a '*downward' spiral of dis-stress.*

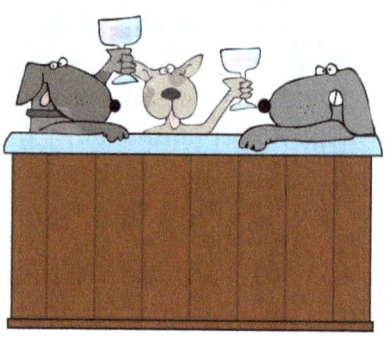

Calming down this Canine Conan, instantly disconnects the drain on all other organs, especially Spleen, resulting in the body being able to process and deal with the stress in a more effective way – an '*upward' spiral to calm*.

TW chills out, it becomes objective rather than subjective and you release its radiant character and it stops draining the entire body. It begins to support it rather than sabotage it. You turn the destructive into the constructive. Canine Conan becomes the Andrex puppy.

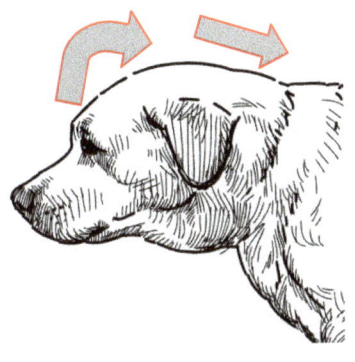

* Using both hands, either flat palms or fingers of your choice (remember the yin and yang discussion previously?). Stroke along from between the eyes up over the forehead, up over the head to the top of her neck(i.e. where her collar would sit).
* Return to your start point and now use the palm of your hand so you take in the sides of her face too
* Massage both ear flaps both inside and out, including the little bud chakras.
* Come back above the eye and very gentle hold just above the eyes.

You can further calm the dog by doing the above and continuing down the outside of the shoulders, down the front legs and off the paws.

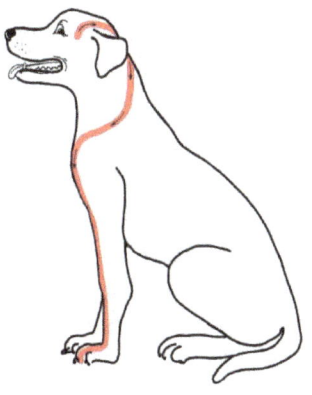

You are tracing *backwards* the entire TW pathway of energy and this will totally calm her Canine Conan, taking it out of 'red alert' and allowing a calm to return in which the body can cope with the perceived stress with grace.

Energy Medicine For Your Dog

At this point, I want to share a story with you.

I was walking my dog Magnus, when another dog attacked and bit him in the face, his left eye was literally hanging out and he was in total dis-stress – his Inner Warrior was running around in a definite and justified state of frightened frenzy. This was truly a survival issue and Conan was doing his job.

I was in the middle of the countryside so it was going to take some time to get him to a vet and I had to walk for about twenty minutes to get to the road.

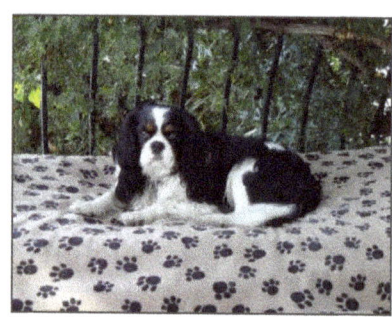

Two things happened:

1. *I carried a 10 kilo dog on one forearm (the other one was cradling his face) over rough terrain for 20 minutes with a strength I didn't realise I possessed. With hindsight it was remarkable, no pain in my knees, wrist, arm or anywhere. It may not have been equal to lifting a truck off a child (which is often used to illustrate a mother's love) but although my arm nearly fell off the next day, during the event it held firm. My inner Xena the Warrior Princess was firing on all cylinders.*

2. *Magnus was in a total state of stress and shock. I could feel him beginning to slip away into unconsciousness as my friend drove me to the*

vet. I wanted to work his energy but both my hands were occupied holding him safely. I did the above stroking (backwards on Triple Warmer) **with my mind** *and a bundle of love. Every now and again figure 8'ing his temples (other TW balancing points). While Triple Warmer is really useful in life-threatening situations, I sensed it had gone from being constructive into a destructive cycle of weakening the other energies, inappropriate over-reaction was dominant.*

He came back into full consciousness within seconds. I had to do this several times, but I kept him conscious and got him to the vet who, while he couldn't save his eye, saved his life – what a brave little soul.

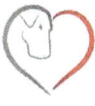

So, the morale of this story is: **Don't underestimate the profound power of your thoughts and love.**

3 POINT MAGIC

You will be holding some powerfully calming acupressure points and visualising at the same time.

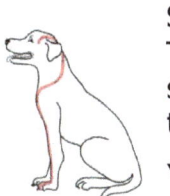

Stroke from her brow all the way down Triple Warmer to her front paws (both sides at the same time) – do this three times. Talk to her and smile.

You choose the visualisation you feel would most benefit her: peace, loving cuddles, curled up on bed, walking happily in a river (that's Mabel's favourite) – think it in glorious colour, with sounds and smells.

At the same time hold 3 points with your fingertips. Keep holding until she breaks away.

The points to hold are:

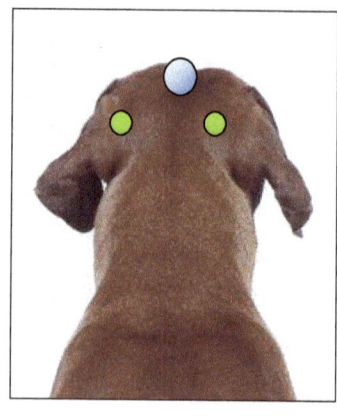

Gallbladder 20, also known as Wind Pond.

It is on *both sides* of the head just below the back of the head halfway between the spine and the base of the ear.

The third point is Governing 20 which is known in Chinese medicine as the Meeting Point of 100 points and is a master point to rebalance energies as a whole. Right on the top of the head.

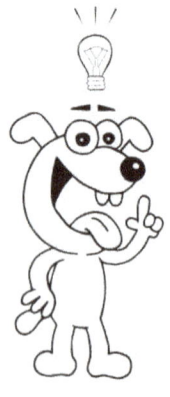

Become Alpha Female, the 'boss', do it through actions rather than aggression; by behaviour rather than vocabulary.

More than 20 years ago I went to a lecture by an amazing man. John Fisher. He founded a website you might find interesting www.apdt.co.uk Association of Pet Dog Trainers. He also wrote a couple of books that I find invaluable and revisit often:

Energy Medicine For Your Dog

THINK DOG – an owner's guide to canine psychology
WHY DOES MY DOG... ?

Both really teach you the language your dog is talking and enable you to communicate in a way he understands. For example:

* Sit on the dog's bed occasionally to make the statement that YOU can go anywhere and that it is not exclusively hers, she has to share it with you as you share your space with her

* Eat before the dog – even if you pretend. *You* are pack leader and that's what pack leaders do in the wild

* Don't let her go through the door or run up the stairs in front of you. It's not cute, it's pack leader behaviour and she is NOT pack leader

* Don't play 'strength' games such as tug-of-war, it encourages a challenge

* Make sure she moves out of your way, don't just step over her

* Encourage her to 'earn' any treats, even if it's a simple 'sit'

* Make eye contact and stand up straight when giving a command. If you bend over she'll think you want to play and won't take you seriously.

* Communicate through eye contact, body language, tone of voice, your behaviour and actions

How to lick your dog!

(MUMMY LICK THAT IS)

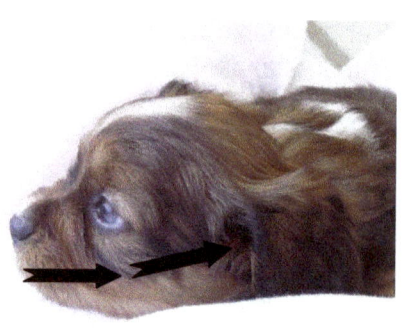

You are simply imitating what her mum did when she was born and in her first few days. With the tips of your fingers stroke from just below the nose, along the side of the mouth then to the ear, pushing gently back as if your fingers were a tongue and come off the ear.

You can do one side at a time or both together.

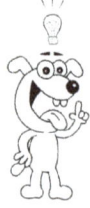

> Your dog's hearing catches ultrasonic, which ours can't. Such remarkable hearing helped their ancestors hunt efficiently.

DOGGIE ELEMENTALS

One of my favourite aspects of human energy medicine is the 5 Elements. It is the system upon which is based the entire philosophy of Traditional Chinese Medicine. It evolved and emerged after hundreds of years of sheer observation. There are 5 different 'stages' of energy and they have been called: 5 Rhythms, 5 Elements, 5 seasons, 5 phases, 5 transformations depending upon which school of TCM you study.

The basic premise is that we (and dogs) are a complex mix and balance of each of these 5 elements and it is an 'energetic dance' to keep them in a harmonious state, as they react to the stresses and pressures of life.

The other aspect is that while we are a mix of all five, there will be one (with sometimes a second element close on its heels) that will be our 'life element', it will be the one that is dominant throughout our entire life, so we could call ourselves an 'Earth Element' person or a 'Wood Element' person etc., we will still plug into the other elements but, especially in times of stress, our primary element will be the one that dictates how we react.

It can be very useful to determine what 'element' your pet is: it will give you an indication of her weaknesses, strengths (both emotionally and physically) and how she reacts and therefore how to communicate most effectively with her. There is no simple test to identify her element, but as you get to know the system in more detail you will probably have an 'ah ha' moment and recognise your pooch.

If you would like to study the elements in more depth there are many very good books[6] out there or email me and I can send you some notes from my 5 Element workshop that you might find interesting.

The 5 elements are:

WATER – WOOD – FIRE – EARTH – METAL

I think the best way to illustrate each of the 5 elements in animals, is to talk about my own pets past and present:

---

[6] Vicki Holme Matthews has a very interesting blog – www.5faces.wordpress.com

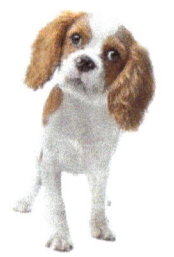

Let's start with Harley, a typical **Water Element**: A Blenheim Cavalier King Charles Spaniel. Harley is lean and fluid, he could get a touch of doggie depression and sink down into the depths of his bed and not want to move, if he could, he'd pull up the duvet and cut out the world. However, I can always tempt him out with something novel, he loves beginning something new. He gets excited running for the ball but then can't really be bothered to see it through and bring it back. He can be quite fearful and jumps when the doorbell goes, is there some hideous canine monster lurking behind the door? He likes salty cat food instead of his own and is always drinking. His weak area is kidney and bladder, so I work a lot on keeping those energies moving and balanced. Another fairly obvious clue is that he loves swimming. When he is quiet and happy at the end of the day, there is a deep wisdom in the depths of his eyes.

Kinmar is a German Shepherd and **Wood** through and through. What a temper, you have to earn his respect and then he is the kindest most loyal of companions, but will switch off if you waffle, he responds to clear, concise commands. He'll defend you against anything, anywhere. He hates being on the lead and prefers to be free and in control

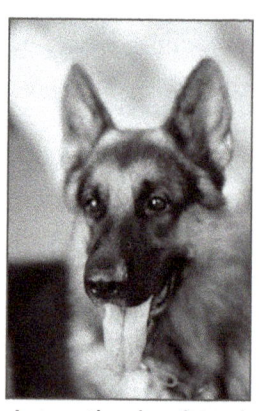

of where he goes and when. If he is on the lead and he meets another dog he will lunge and bark as if doing that gives the impression that HE is in control. This is done to assure that things don't get 'out of control' which is really what upsets a Wood. Don't mess with him when he is eating. As he gets older he is getting less flexible in his joints and more rigid in his thinking too. He likes to get things done so when you pick up the lead, you had better walk him rather than dawdle around finding your keys – *'come on Mum let's do it and do it now!'*.

Liver and Gallbladder are the organs to take care of with Kinmar, he often suffers itchy, red eyes and as Gallbladder is associated with outwardly directed anger, he can be rather grumpy!

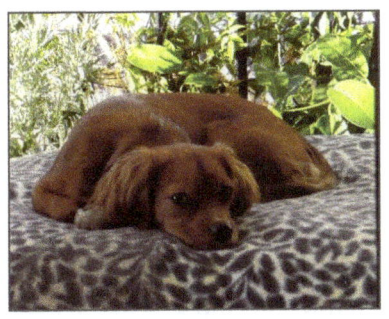

MABEL – a Cavalier King Charles and 'mutt' cross – she has a red coat and is a very definite **Fire Element** – the red should be a clue here. What else?

She loves everyone, everyone basks in her charisma. She is very loving and loves being fussed over. She makes everyone feel they are her very best friend. She lives totally in the present moment. Training her was a challenge in itself, she wants to please but boy oh boy does she want to have fun too and you can guess which wins out. Keeping her attention as her mind flits from one thing to another is a feat of patience. However, you have to laugh and feel the pure joy of her experiencing life. When I pick up the lead she is like Zebedee jumping in the air with joy and excitement. I need to watch she doesn't get over stressed or anxious, when she does she barks hysterically until she can hardly breathe. The vet checks her heart every year to ensure there are no problems. Fire governs Heart, Small Intestine, Pericardium (which protects the heart) and Triple Warmer (the flow of energy associated with stress, the Canine Conan mentioned in this book).

MAGNUS – a Tricolour Cavalier King Charles – so **Earth** it warms your heart. Always wanting to please you and making sure you are happy; an absolute joy to train – we even got past advanced training and onto agility. It was so easy to train him as he loves his grub and is easily bribed! Loving his food causes a slight rotund aspect to this young man (didn't I say

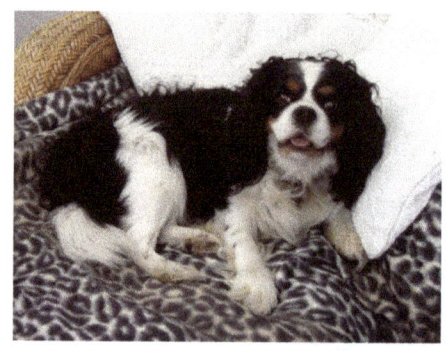

dogs reflect their owners). He adores walking in the hills but is always mindful of me and where I am, sensitive to my needs, protective and caring. Even when he doesn't want to go out, he will, just to make me happy. He is perhaps happiest at home, on my lap. He can be a worry wart and have problems with metabolising change of any kind. He likes routine and the predictable. I keep a close eye on his Stomach and Spleen (immunity).

MUMKIN is **Metal** through and through, fine boned and beautiful she is totally aloof, no running around in excited circles for her. She likes her bowls in alignment, her meals on time – all very precise and organised. If she was a human she would have a 'checklist',

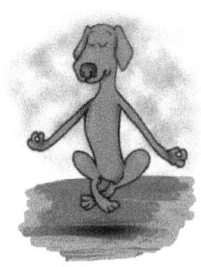

alphabetically sorted and colour coded. Pretty low down on that checklist would be stroking and cuddles, under no circumstances must you attempt either of these unless she asks for them, then you have to drop everything and attend to her needs and consider yourself lucky to be able to perform such a sacred duty and you had better do it properly not half heartedly or she will fix you with one of her disdainful stares.

This is one madam who doesn't mind if you leave her alone. She is mistress of canine meditation. She likes to ruminate, cogitate and otherwise process what is going on around her, before making her mind up on a course of action. Ultimately she likes to be in charge and stands strong as steel until she is.

As Metal rules lung and large intestine, she sometimes has problems with her elimination or respiratory tract.

Actually, I'll come clean, Mumkin is my cat, I simply have never owned a metal dog, it seems to go against the canine personality in general: But, they must exist – is yours one?

Do you recognise your dog in any of these?

- ❋ WATER – she will respond to new and creative activities
- ❋ WOOD – you'll have to establish yourself as alpha dog
- ❋ FIRE – just make it fun with lots of action and cuddles
- ❋ EARTH – let her know you need her, not too much change in one go and keep a bag of treats in your pocket
- ❋ METAL – they are in charge - just do what you're told!

A simple way to balance the elements in your dog is to:

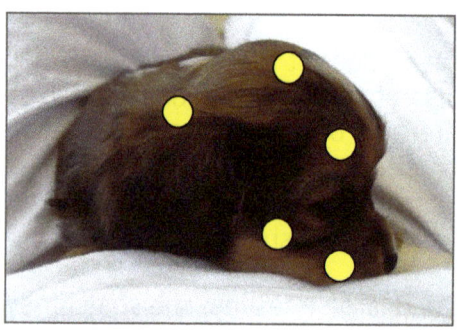

One hand holds the

Points above the eyes, top of head and back of head.

Keep one hand on these points and with the other hold one side of the face so you get in the point on the 'cheek' and by the eye. After a minute, release that hand and hold the other side.

Just hold for a few seconds when she is quiet and it brings into balance all the Elements by stimulating key neurovascular holding points that in turn balance out each meridian and element.

You may like to talk or think as you hold these points:

- *May you know the wisdom of your ancestors*
- *May you be flexible in mind and body*
- *May you know joy*
- *May you feel safe and loved*
- *May you let go of any sadness you have felt.*

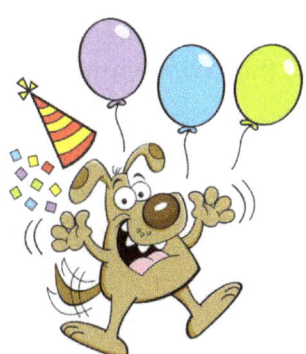

TRACING SOME VERY STRANGE FLOWS

I love these strange ancient flows of energy and they translate beautifully on our dogs.

Little is known here in the West but they are used extensively in TCM [Traditional Chinese Medicine] in the East. They appear to predate meridians and are the first energy circuit to appear in the developing foetus – they are truly ancient flows of energy that perhaps, in our distant ancestors, flowed freely through the body, some, over time however, repeatedly began to serve specific organs – was it these that then developed into what we know as the fixed energy channels called meridians? *Are meridians just Strangeflows stuck in a rut?*

Dogs are far more connected to their 'strange flows' than us humans and respond quickly to working with them; they appreciate that these flows are flows connected to 'joy' and feel good. They generate joy in your life.

They help your dog deal with change, they protect using the principle of harmony (They are diplomats not 'special forces') and will troubleshoot anywhere in the body where help is needed. So you can begin to see how very useful these flows can be in maintaining your dog's well being.

Your dog may be a pampered pooch or a rescue rascal – both will benefit from free flowing Strangeflows. As you will, and that's the beauty of working this technique, as you balance her flows, yours react too and begin to find their own harmony.

One very simple way of activating the flows is to lightly scratch your dog's back all over, from top to bottom and lots of figure 8's both on the back and anywhere on the body. This will instantly activate all the flows.

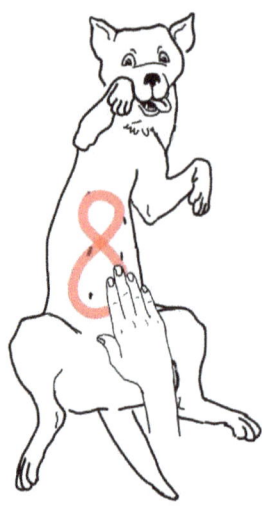

Remember when you were a child you drew letters on you friends' backs and they had to guess what you had written? Children all over the world do this. Why? Because instinctively they know it makes them feel more joyful.

You can also 'trace' the flows. Rub your hands together and shake off any stale and tired energy and place them over the beginning of the flow and slowly move your hands along it. Keeping to the direction indicated until you reach the end. Do on both sides of the body.

Your hands are like little electromagnetic pads and when you align them with intent to a flow on your pet, as you move the hand, the energy on the flow will follow. So you will literally be moving your pet's energy with your hands.

Follow the diagrams below for my 2 favourite flows.

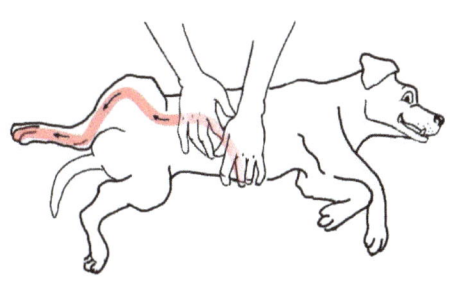

Belt flow – with your dog on her back, pull round the 'waist' a couple of times before tracing down and off the opposite leg and paw. Repeat on the other side. This flow is vital for your dog's ability to balance her natural instincts and the practicalities of being your pet! Good for hip and leg health and a must for digestion and reproductive systems.

Here's one of the most valuable 'tracings' you can do on your dog (and on yourself for that matter). It's called Regulator. That's exactly what it does, it helps her regulate and adjust to any change in her life or any change you are trying to achieve with your work on her.

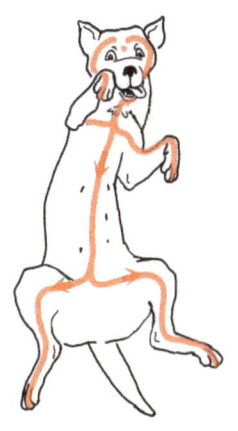

* Start with your hands on her third eye

* Trace round her face to the tip of her jaw

- Down over her windpipe to her throat
- Branch out to the shoulders
- Down both legs hands around the limbs and off front paws
- Hands off and place on her chest
- Down the front of the belly
- Off both her back paws and give them a little squeeze

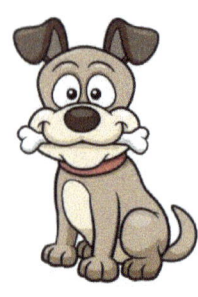

WORKING WITH THE PATHWAYS OF ENERGY

Meridians are electromagnetic pathways running through your dog's body, along which energy flows. They all link together and you can influence and balance them very easily by 'tracing' them with an open palm (as described in the section above). Most are on both sides of the body, so always work on them both.

Each meridian is associated with a specific organ/system and influences defined emotions. Tracing brings energy into the pathway, strengthening it to help restore an energetic harmony that in turn helps your dog heal both emotionally and physically.

Meridian pathways can give you vital clues when things begin to go wrong, either on an emotional or physical level.

You can test each one (with a surrogate) by holding the easiest end point (normally on a paw) and testing.

Follow the suggested sequence, if you fall out of sequence no harm will come to your dog. We suggest this sequence as where one pathway 'ends' the next one starts so you can think of it as one long continuous flow.

Reset the meridian by running your open hand backwards along it once and forwards 3 times. Work 1" off the body. This has the effect of taking it back to 'default' by taking out old stale, tired energy (the backward motion) and bringing in fresh clean energy (the forward motion).

Do not get too obsessed about the exact route, you are not going to be putting acupuncture needles into the meridian. You will be using your open palm and lashings of intention and love which will be enough for you to make a positive impact on the meridian energy.

If in doubt, retest after the 'reset' and you will find it now tests strong.

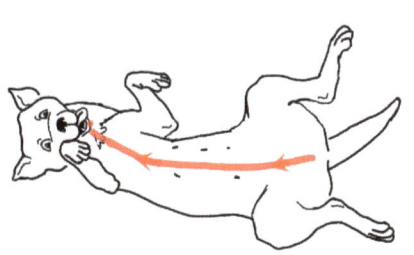

CENTRAL MERIDIAN

Starts near the anus area and runs straight up the centre of the body to the lower lip.

GOVERNING MERIDIAN

Also starts near the anus (you can start at the root of the tail on the back) and runs straight up the back, over the top of the head and ends on the upper lip.

We naturally brush backwards on this meridian; remember to do one last stroke, in the energy field from tail to head to ensure the meridian is strong.

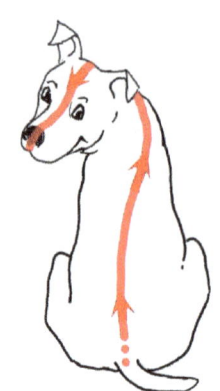

STOMACH MERIDIAN

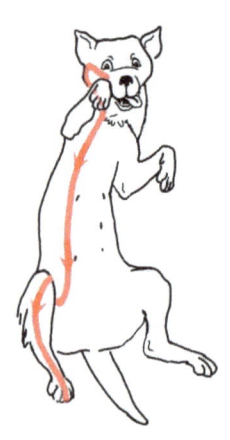

- start just below each eye
- drop straight down to the jaw
- along the jaw and up to the front of the ear
- straight down the underside of the neck, chest, abdomen
- flare out at the hips and down the front of the hind legs. come off the 2nd toe.

ON BOTH SIDES OF THE BODY

SPLEEN MERIDIAN

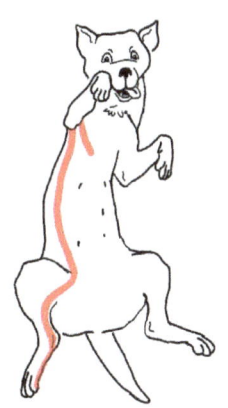

* Starts on the medial toe of the back leg

* Up the inside of the hind leg to abdomen

* Up over the abdomen up to the 'armpit' and down to mid ribs

ON BOTH SIDES OF THE BODY

HEART MERIDIAN

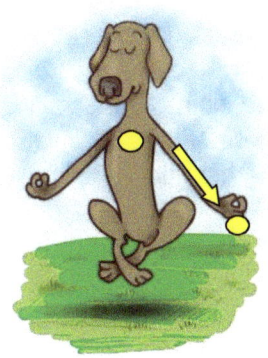

* Starts over the heart area

* Runs down the chest

* Down the inside of the front leg

* Ends coming off the lateral (4th) toe

ON BOTH SIDES OF THE BODY

SMALL INTESTINE

- Outside of the lateral 4th toe
- Up along back of leg
- Over the shoulder blade
- To the bottom of the neck
- Along neck to jawbone
- Up cross the cheek
- Past the eye
- Ends just in front of the ear

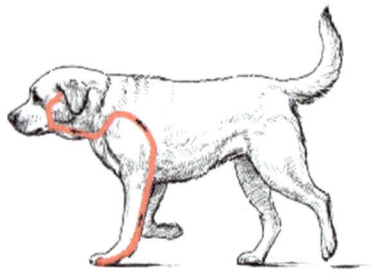

ON BOTH SIDES OF THE BODY

BLADDER MERIDIAN

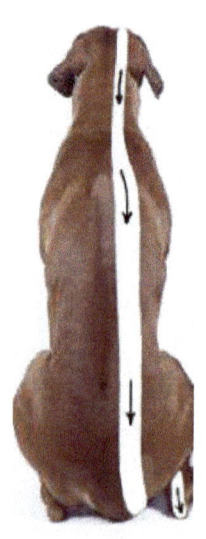

- Begins between the eyes
- Comes up over the skull
- Down back of neck to shoulder blade
- Spread palm out so it covers a dual pathway down the side of the spine
- Becomes one again at the pelvis
- Runs down the back of the hind leg
- At the 'heel' comes round to the outside
- Comes off the outside of the 4th toe (back leg)

ON BOTH SIDES OF THE BODY

KIDNEY MERIDIAN

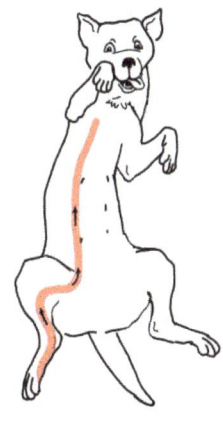

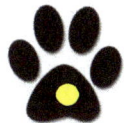

Begins under to paw
Runs up inside leg
Up the abdomen
Up the chest
Ends at base of the neck

ON BOTH SIDES OF THE BODY

CIRCULATION SEX PERICARDIUM

- Starts at the chest area near the heart
- Runs down to the elbow
- Down inside of foreleg
- Come off the 2nd toe

ON BOTH SIDES OF THE BODY

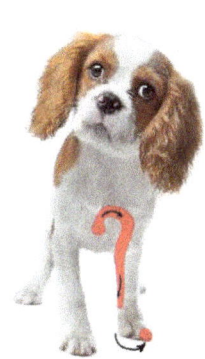

TRIPLE WARMER

* Begins at outside of the 4th toe (front leg)
* Runs up the leg to elbow
* Over the shoulder
* Up the side of the neck
* Behind the ear
* Over top of ear
* Ends at temples/side of eye

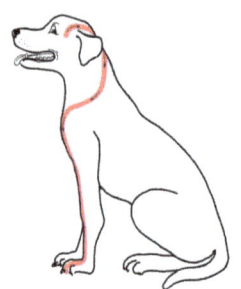

BOTH SIDES OF THE BODY

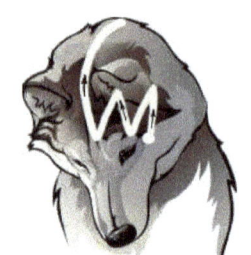

GALLBLADDER

* Starts at the outside corner of the eye
* Move back to the ear
* Move forward to the temples
* Move back over the ear
* Move forward
* over the forehead
* Back on the forehead
* Down the neck
* Down to the shoulder
* Over the side of the body to the pelvic area
* Down the outside of the back leg
* Comes off 2nd toe

BOTH SIDES OF THE BODY

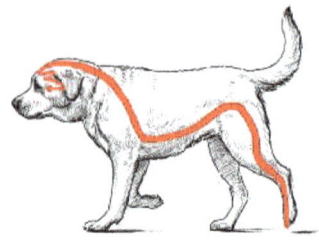

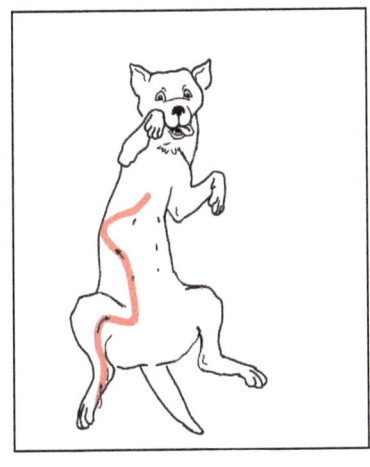

LIVER MERIDIAN

* Begins at the dew claw on back leg
* Runs up the inside of the leg to pelvic area
* Fares out to the side
* Comes back in and meets at lower chest area

BOTH SIDES OF THE BODY

LUNG

* Starts over the lung area
* Runs down inside of front leg
* Ends coming off the due claw

BOTH SIDES OF THE BODY

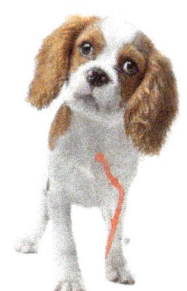

LARGE INTESTINE

* Tip of the 1st toe (medial) of front leg
* Up the inside of the leg
* Move out to the elbows
* Up over front of shoulder
* Up side of neck
* Along top lip
* Ends at side of nostril

BOTH SIDES OF THE BODY

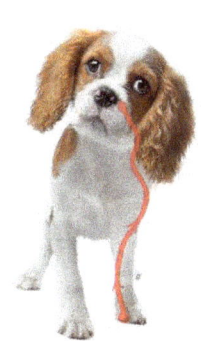

Energy Medicine For Your Dog

Every pathway is associated with a 2 hour time 'slot' – does that time slot correspond to a physical symptom or behavioural quirk of your dog? If it does then maybe by balancing the associated meridian you can influence the physical or emotional aspects.

Also, where does the physical problem occur? What meridian is it on? Try working with that meridian (by working with, I mean resetting the meridian as described above: tracing backwards x 1 forwards x 3) and see if it helps.

We need flow around the 'Meridian Wheel, with no blockages; when they do occur the energy becomes stagnant and tired and can cause problems. Pain is always associated with stagnant energies.

By regularly tracing your dog's meridians you can help prevent things moving into the physical from the energetic and if there is already a physical problem, by getting the energy moving you are allowing space for the dog's inner healer to function to her optimum level.

Let's take an example:

Say Magnus has a stiff back leg and hip area. First of all, what is stiffness associated with? Wood element. So I would immediately suspect Wood (liver and gallbladder).

I can then look at what meridian runs through or close to the painful area and in this case it would be gallbladder on the outside and Liver on the inside leg (in another example it might be another element) – so I would definitely be balancing Gallbladder and Liver. I might look for further clues, has Magnus been more grumpy lately? Remember GB is associated with outwardly directed 'anger'. Does it get worse at a particular time of day? In the case of Wood I would be looking at 11pm – 3am. I might also suspect Bladder, Stomach, Kidney and Spleen which also all run through the back legs.

I might therefore surrogate test the suspect meridians by holding the end point of each (see list above), focussing with my mind on the route it takes and testing. Don't worry if you are not quite sure of the spot, intention is king in energy medicine. Energy follows intention (and your hand).

If a meridian tests 'weak'; **reset and retest** – it should now test strong.

If it doesn't, then trace the meridian and test – if it is still weak that could indicate that the pathway has TOO much energy on it, it definitely didn't want the extra energy you were bringing in by tracing. It will however benefit from tracing BACKWARDS on it. So, do that and test – it should now be strong as you have taken some of that over energy out and restored it to a balanced flow and you have one happy meridian.

An energy pathway can either have TOO MUCH energy or TOO LITTLE energy flowing along it. Testing identifies there is a problem but does not define if it is over or under energised. Therefore always retest after you trace: if it's strong then great, it needed a bit of extra energy. However, if it is still weak then the chances are that you need to take some energy out by tracing backwards on the flow.

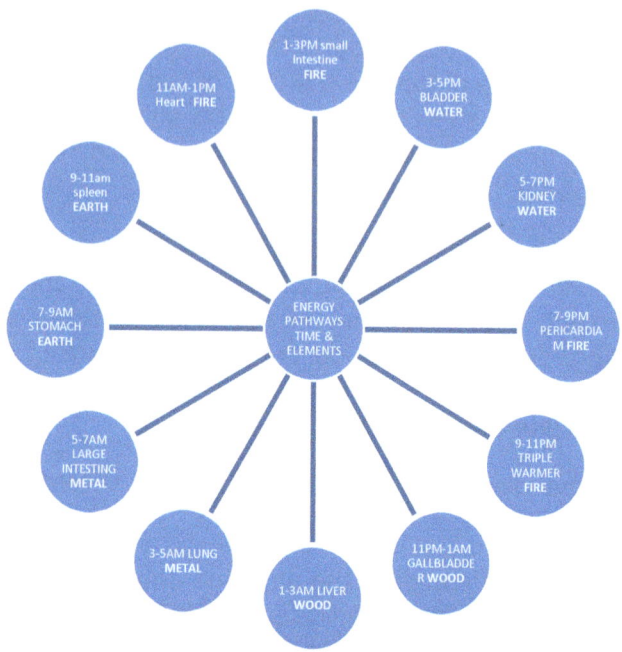

It is worth noting that pain is nearly always associated with too much energy which has inevitably become stagnant. Remove that excess energy, new energy comes in and moves and the pain moves too.

Keywords associated with each meridian:

Central	Affects all the Yin meridians: lung, spleen, heart, kidney, Circ Sex and Liver. How she interacts with the world around her
Governing	Affects all the Yang meridians: Stomach, Large Intestine, Small Intestine, Bladder, Triple Warmer and Gallbladder.

Energy Medicine For Your Dog

	We naturally brush backwards on Governing – head to tail, this does no harm as we do it with love. However, if you are specifically balancing the meridians, ensure you end on Governing in the correct direction – tail to head. As this does go against the direction of the hair growth you can work just off the body.
	Courage + anything to do physically with the spine
Stomach	Obsessive worry and digestion
Spleen	Her immunity + over submissiveness
Heart	Sadness (they do feel it).
Small Intestine	Indecisiveness and digestion
Bladder	Fear, hopelessness (rescue animals) spinal and urinary health
Kidney	Fearfulness
Circ Sex	Anxious alienation
Triple Warmer	That Inner Warrior in a frenzy!
Gallbladder	Outwardly directed anger and aggression
Liver	Irritability and flexibility of both mind and body
Lung	Depression, grief and of course, anything to do with breathing.
Large Intestine	Difficulty in letting go, elimination of waste + any skin problems

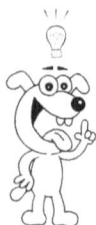

Dogs respond more to positive rather than negative commands: 'quiet' rather than 'don't bark'.

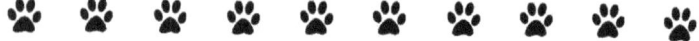

TO SUMMARISE THE END POINTS ON THE PADS:

Front legs

- THE EQUIVALENT OF OUR THUMB (dew claw) – lung
- Forefinger (medial) – Large Intestine
- Middle finger – Pericardium
- Ring finger – Triple Warmer
- Little finger – Heart and Small Intestine

Back legs

- Central pad – Kidney
- Medial 1st Spleen and Liver
- 2nd – Stomach
- 3rd – Gallbladder
- 4th Bladder

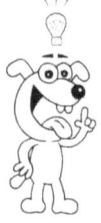

It is said to ease the grief of a pet that has lost its owner or companion, let her see and sniff the body. It will then more easily accept the death and not suffer the confusion and frustration of waiting for its companion to return.

HOW TO BUILD HER IMMUNITY

There are two systems that are your dog's best friend with regard to her immunity:

- the lymph system
- Spleen energy.

Let's take the Lymph system first as we have already addressed it with the Spinal Flush and massage (above) the former stimulates the system via the reflex points along the spine, the latter encouraging the elimination of toxins and of course regular exercise is as essential to your dog as it is to you, to get lymph moving around the body and encouraging toxic removal.

The more toxins removed the less stress on the body which results in energy being free to patrol, repair and replenish.

Specific acupressure points to boost her immune system include:

Hold each of these points for at least 30 seconds. The hold should be gentle, yet firm, using your fingertips. Hold on both sides of the body. On humans we seek to feel a 'pulse' when holding points, you may be able to do this with your dog, but often it can be difficult, so hold the intention of strengthening her Inner Healer.

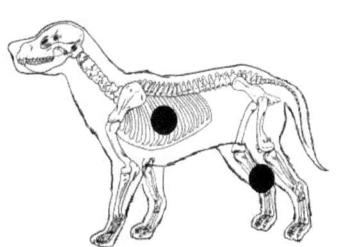

Spleen 6 – on the inside of the back leg just above the (knee) joint.

Spleen 21 – on her side, half way along her ribs.

You can trace and reset her Spleen meridian (on both sides), gently with an open palm. Go backwards once and forwards 3 times. Don't go against the grain of her hair growth, lighten up the pressure of your touch so it doesn't annoy her.

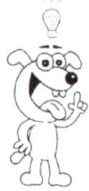

> Don't let her sleep near any electrical equipment; the energies these appliances emit are not conducive to health. Be careful with household chemicals too, they can provoke a reaction.

THE IDEAL DOGGIE DIET

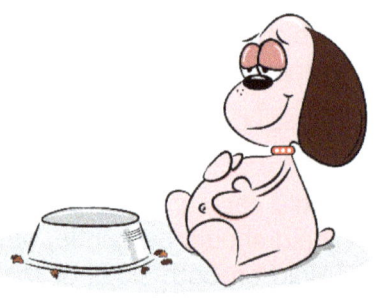

This could be one of the most valuable tools in your canine care kit. Eating to suit your dog's body chemistry (which is unique as a thumbprint), enhances her immunity and helps maintain health and well-being in general. Most skin problems will respond to a change in diet as will a behavioural problem.

Learn to surrogate test, which if you have never done it 'reads' complicated but is really so easy once you take the time to practice and become confident. I promise you, the only thing that stands between you and an accurate energy test is _you_. Once you relax and stop judging yourself or feeling you can't do it or comparing yourself to the Donna Eden's of this world... then you'll suddenly find – hey! It works! And you are off and running.

Simply test what you plan to feed your dog. If it tests weak then don't feed it to her that day. If it tests strong then feed it to her, confident that her body will absorb the nutrition and eliminate the waste just as Nature intended with no undue stress. She will not be squandering her energy on processing foods that conflict with her chemistry, that energy is freed to perform maintenance and repair duties of the body in general.

You may choose the dried food, the wet food or the home prepared route – whichever, and all have their merits – **_test before she ingests._**

You will need a third person, a surrogate, who effectively acts as an 'energy receiving station'; they will be the link between you and your dog. This may sound unbelievable, but it works.

All the testing is carried out in the normal way on the surrogate, (basic guidelines to testing at the back of the book). The surrogate and dog maintain contact throughout. This contact is most normally a hand on shoulder or head/neck.

Needless to say it is imperative that the surrogate is in balance so that they can act as an effective connection. A simple balance of 3 Thumps and X Crawl is often all that is necessary (see at the end of the book).

Check the surrogate is testing correcting by getting them to make a false statement and energy test it – it should be weak. Energy test a true statement and it should be strong. You know the energy is talking to you and in the right way.

Energy Medicine For Your Dog

Statements would be something simple and straightforward:

> 🐾 *My name is Minnie Mouse*
> 🐾 *My name is Maddie King*

So the basic surrogate routine would be...

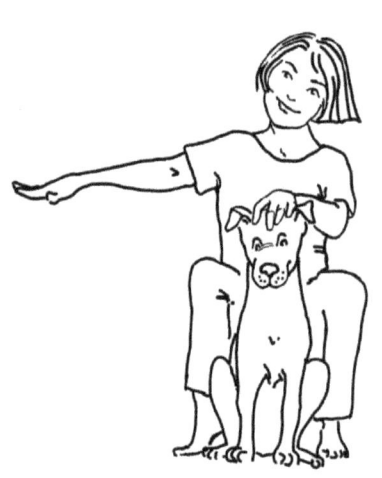

- *Balance yourself with basic 3 thumps*
- *Surrogate does the same*
- *Energy test the surrogate to ensure they are in balance and you can get a clear test*
- *Surrogate places hand on the dog. They can be standing or sitting, it doesn't matter.*
- *Both of you to be grounded and bring the intention of testing the dog.*
- *You introduce the substance being tested anywhere against the dog and test the surrogate (if this is difficult, you can hold the substance against the surrogate with clear intention).*
- *If you want to **test a meridian,** simply hold one of the end points on the paws.*
- *If you want to **test a chakra**, tap over the chakra and test.*

Grab a friend, grab your dog and have a go.

> *You can energy test most things via a surrogate. If you would like more details on energy testing yourself and others email me and I can send you information. I want to keep it really simple for this book and not confuse or muddy the waters with excessive details.*

Keep a record as the memory can be selective. You will be surprised at the results. I have done workshops on food testing for your pet and have taken along every conceivable sample of dog food (I raided and bribed all the pet stores in Fulham for some of the posh ones and the supermarkets for the cheaper brands, and own brands). Often a cheap 'own' brand would suit her body chemistry better than an expensive brand – for that day. I'm not saying everyone should run out and buy really cheap dog food with dodgy ingredients, but I am saying: **let go of any expectations and test with an open mind** and now and again you will be surprised at the results.

The following foods can cause damage to your dog:

- Grapes
- Raisins
- Chocolate and sugar
- Macadamia nuts
- Onions
- Garlic
- Avocado (although some dogs love them)
- Apple or pear seeds
- Caffeine and alcohol
- Milk and dairy (it's the breast milk of another species and hard to digest)
- Excessive salt

Tall dogs should not eat off the floor. Put their food on a raised surface such as a stool. In the action of putting their heads to the floor to eat, their internal organs move forward and they can get 'bloat' which is a condition where the stomach fills with gas and expands. There are some great adjustable pet feeders on the market now.

One very useful way of surrogate testing food is in relationship to any skin conditions your dog suffers, these can be very frustrating and distressing for both of you. If you faithfully test her food before she ingests, it should help any dry, itchy or inflamed condition improve, if it is caused or exacerbated by food.

Also the techniques that reduce stress will help. It could however be a problem related to something external in the environment – test bedding, household chemicals or anything that springs to mind. Some dogs have been known to react to the water. Energy testing helps you detect the source of the irritation.

Have you ever wondered if you dog might benefit from a canine supplement – such as glucosamine for the joints? Well, if you know how to test you can take the guess work out of it.

* Touch the joints that are stiff and energy test, they will probably test weak.
* Now hold the supplement against the joint and test – is it strong?

If yes, your dog might well benefit from taking that supplement.

I had a very open-minded independent pet shop owner in London and he used to allow me to test supplements in this way before I bought them so I didn't make too many expensive mistakes. If you don't have that luxury, ask if they have any samples. If not use your common sense and buy the smallest bottle.

USING A PENDULUM

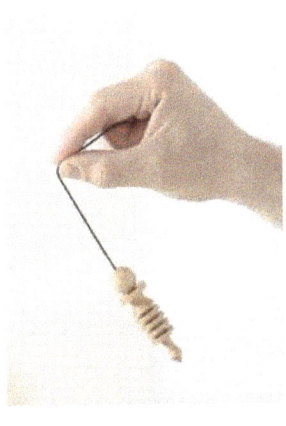

Have you ever pondered upon pendulums. They are neither magic nor 'hocus pocus'. Using them provides a simple and straightforward tool to communicate with your 'inner voice of wisdom' and that of your dog. It is a bridge between your rational and intuitive minds. It allows you to access the wise woman (or sage) deep within you.

We instinctively all know exactly what we need to optimise our health, or that of our loved ones and pets, but that knowledge sometimes gets lost through the demands of contemporary life and the lack of 'instinct' validation as we grow up. A kind of static builds up and you can no longer grasp onto your intuition, it becomes elusive. Like looking at the static on your television set, you know if you could find the right button to press then that 'static' would turn into a clear, vibrant, full colour picture. After you have been using the pendulum for a while, you will begin to observe that your natural instinct and intuition becomes stronger, the static begins to disperse and glimpses of the picture emerge.

Dowsing is still used in some Mediterranean countries to find water, in rural areas especially of France and

Spain, the Water Dowser is part of the community and is sometimes paid by the Town Hall.

What is a pendulum? a simple weight on a thread – the weight may be a cotton reel or a solid gold pendant, large or small, light or heavy, simple or ornate – it is entirely your choice, a ring on the thread, even a teabag on a string will work.

Length of thread: you will need enough to permit movement. A long thread produces a slow, lazy movement that takes its time changing. A shorter thread produces a faster movement. An average length is 9 inches and you may hold anywhere on that 9 inches. I personally hold about 3" up from the pendulum itself.

Prepare yourself: 3 thumps, hook up (see end of book). Get yourself tuned in to your dog.

Nobody really knows how dowsing works; it just seems to and has been successfully used for centuries. Let go of your left brain, rational thoughts and open the door to your more intuitive right brain.

Basic holding: as a true blue beginner, follow these instructions and as you gain confidence you can change any aspect of them to suit your personal style as you discover what works best for you. The elbow should be below the shoulder and the wrist below the elbow. Hold the thread between the thumb and index finger, both pointing down.

Make sure your hands or legs are not crossed or touching each other. Sit with feet apart and firmly planted on the ground.

If you are right handed use your right hand and if left handed use your left. This is a general rule of thumb and if you are drawn to use your less dominant hand, then do so. There is a school of thought that says the less dominant hand is the more intuitive. Experiment and see which way feels and works better for you.

Let's use the chakras as an example of testing. But you could equally hold the pendulum over your dog's joints, spine or organs.

Hold the pendulum over the chakra, bringing all your attention to it. This is not the time to be thinking of what you are going to wear for that hot date on Saturday night or compiling your supermarket shopping list, or trying to remember if you picked up the dry cleaning.

Simply observe what the pendulum does. It should pick up the energy and start swinging (normally in a circle to reflect the flow of energy) in a strong deliberate manner. You are <u>not</u> asking a question you are simply allowing the pendulum to pick up the energy and move to provide an 'illustration' of the strength of the energy.

* If the swing is **strong**, it indicates that the chakra or joint is in good working order.
* If the swing is there but very **sluggish** then the chakra or joint will be sluggish too and will benefit from some energy work.
* If there is **no swing** then the chakra or joint could be chronically 'tired' or stagnant, nothing much is moving. Over time this can cause problems in the associated physical aspects of your dog.

Don't forget the Number 1 rule of energy work

ENERGY MUST MOVE!

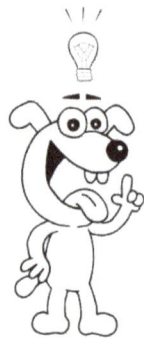

If you are familiar with the work of Dr Emoto you will know that words can influence the molecular structure of water (and we are made up of more than 75% water). On a piece of paper write the words LOVE & GRATITUDE and place it under your dog's water bowl so that she can lap up the energy of those two words, which Dr Emoto found to be the most positive for our health and well being.

Of course if you are a little Virgo like me you will laminate your piece of paper and in fact have several, under the food, the water, in the fridge, under her bed... all over the place – I even have one under my computer on the premise that it can't do any harm, only good!

A CANINE CARE KIT

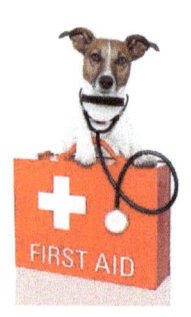

Isn't it the Scouts that say 'always be prepared'? Well you should be prepared on behalf of your dog. Here are a few suggestions of what to keep in your Canine Care Kit.

- Australian Bush Flower Emergency Essence
- Healing Herbs – 5 Flowers

Administer either of these after any shock or trauma. Excellent post surgery. Drops can be straight in her mouth or in a little water and will benefit the entire body.

Topically there are sprays now available. If you want to focus on a particular part of the body, spray on the area. In the event of an injury or wound that is open, you should not put it on directly because of the risk of infection, so spray it on the nearest 'safe' place.

So, for example, when Magnus was bitten, as soon as I got him home (I sadly didn't have it on me when I was walking) I put Emergency Essence in his mouth – closely followed by his favourite treat – remember I said he would do anything for food. I then diluted 20 drops in a small 10 ml spray with water. Shook it up and sprayed about 3" away from the dressing on his eye.

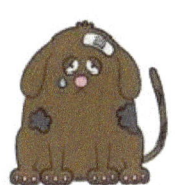

- Aloe Vera – applied topically for cuts or burns. I keep mine in the fridge. I don't know if there is any scientific evidence, but it seems to work better when cold.

- Arnica – applied topically and taken homoeopathically (internally) for any wound, bruise or bite. Again, excellent before and after surgery.

- One small drop of Milk Thistle (tincture) in her water to support her liver if she has to take medication.

- Ginger, add a little to her food to reduce flatulence

- Garlic to repel fleas – they hate it.

- Lemon repels fleas, dilute with water and apply to her coat.

- Fleas don't like mint so put some leaves on her bed.

- Figure 8'ing is a totally free First Aid technique that you can do anywhere: over cuts and bruises especially.

- Mummy Licks extended up and over the ear is the other useful technique to take your pet out of inappropriate stress response.

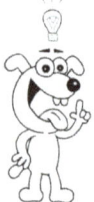

Kick start her energy by massaging the main pad on each front paw. This is Kidney 1 where the entire meridian energy system starts.

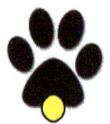

FLOWER ESSENCES

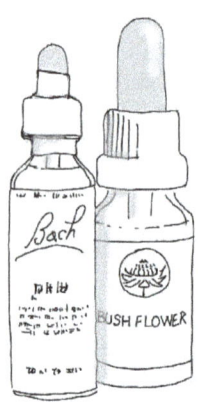

Flower essences are easy, safe and effective, in fact animals can respond more quickly to them than humans do. They will support, on an emotional level, any treatment your dog is receiving or help her through an emotional upset (e.g. firework night or separation anxiety).

There are now myriad essences available. My two personal favourites are:

- The Australian Bush Flower Remedies[7]
- Healing Herbs[8]

There is nothing new about these flower essences. Flowers and plants have been used since the beginning of time by healers of all cultures. Every flower and plant has a specific vibrational energy that can influence your dog in a subtle, safe and positive way.

These essences capture that energy in a 'homeopathic' liquid form. The plant or flower is picked at dawn (the zenith of their vitality) and placed in water, in the sunlight, for several hours. The liquid is then strained and forms the base of the Essence. It has no actual molecules of the plant or flower and as such not to be confused with herbal tinctures.

Adding a few drops to your dog's drinking water will begin to balance out her emotions and energy. 7 drops in a normal dog bowl and a few more if your dog is huge and less if she is tiny. Be reassured that they are <u>self-adjusting</u> and as such whatever dose you administer, no harm will come to your dog. Very occasionally, there may be a mini 'healing crisis' as emotions come to the surface, but this should pass very quickly (within 24 hours).

You can use a surrogate to test which flower essence is needed. Simply hold the essence against the dog's body and test the surrogate (who will be connected via her other hand to your dog):

---

[7] www.ausflowers.com.au

[8] <u>www.healingherbs.co.uk</u> this is a company that backs Dr Bach remedies in the 'old fashioned' way and to a high quality.

 Energy Medicine For Your Dog

- ❖ If the test is weak, then don't use it.
- ❖ If the test is strong then it could either be 'neutral' or strengthening to your dog. To determine which:
- ❖ Weaken the surrogate by tracing down from mouth to pelvic area. Repeat the test.
- ❖ If it's weak then the essence is neutral, it won't do any harm but neither will it strengthen your dog. It's a signal to seek another essence or route up the mountainside of healing.
- ❖ However if it now tests strong then voila! It has the power to strengthen that weak muscle and is therefore going to have a positive impact on your dog.

Keep your feet on the ground and objectively evaluate your dog's behaviour and health over the next couple of weeks. Observe and see if there is an improvement or subtle shift. Don't fall foul to ENCS *(Emperor's New Clothing Syndrome)*

Essences can be obtained easily online nowadays either direct or from one of my favourite sites www.nutricentre.com

If you feel your dog is responding well, you might like to research in more depth with either of these companies.

www.healingherbs.co.uk – I choose this company because it was started by a single person in 1988 who wanted to keep it small and prepare the essences with total integrity. Julian Barnard is still involved in every step of the process. If you would like more details about Dr Bach and the remedies, there is an educational section on the site with many free videos, he has been very generous with his information.

www.ausflowers.com.au – is the main site with distributors in the UK. Ian White set up ABFE and has also kept his hand firmly on the rudder. I find they nearly always test strong on clients – find the right one and they really make a difference.

You might like to make up your own (very easy and you don't necessarily have to dance naked under a full moon!) – It's all about intention.

Here are a few that might interest you:

The essences in *italics* are Australian Bush and in normal typeface are Healing Herbs.

Black Eyed Susan	*Is THE stress and anxiety essence for dogs. Also good for irritability.*	*Sundew*	*To help your dog focus*
Chicory	For the dog who is over-possessive of his owner, is always seeking attention and is unhappy being left along.	Walnut or *Bottlebrush*	To help her cope with change. So great for if you are moving house
Dog Rose	*For the fearful or shy dog. Often will bark or howl.*	*Flannel Flower*	*For the dog that doesn't like to be touched. Try some before grooming or a massage.*
Holly *Mountain Devil*	*For the jealous, suspicious dog who is always barking. For dogs who have suffered past abuse. Especially good if you are...*	Aspen	*For a nervous dog especially in unfamiliar surroundings*

	trying to introduce a second dog/puppy into the home. Or if the owner is having a baby.		
Impatiens	For the impatient, irritable dog	Chestnut	If she has had harsh early training + helps with training and learning. Helps break bad habits.
Mimulus	For the dog who is always fearful of the slightest sound or movement. This is the one to use when you KNOW what she is afraid of.	Honeysuckle	If you suspect your dog will miss you while he is in kennels. Or if you are inheriting an animal from someone who has had to move on.
Star of Bethlehem	Perfect for rescue dogs. Trauma, grief, injury or abuse.	Vervain Or Crowea	*Will calm down a hyped up, over stresed dog.*
Vine and Beech combined	2 drops of each. Vine is for domination and Beech for intolerance. Good in groups where hierarchy and dominance may be an issue.	Olive	For the exhausted dog
Gymea Lily	*Posture, aching bones, spinal alignment*	*Boronia*	*Obsessive behaviour / habits*

And of course, the classic Dr Bach Rescue Remedy, 5 Flowers or the ABFE Emergency Essence are all essentials in a time of trauma or shock. Try them out next November 5th – Guy Fawkes Night. Begin administering a couple of hours before the fireworks are due to start.

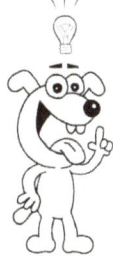

If a dog is truly hostile, don't move a muscle or it will be seen as a challenge. Stand still and sideways onto the dog (frontal approach is a challenge) and then walk away very very slowly. A dog will rarely bark when attacking, so beware the silent snarl.

GOOD VIBRATIONS
ESSENTIAL OILS
NB oils should always be diluted!

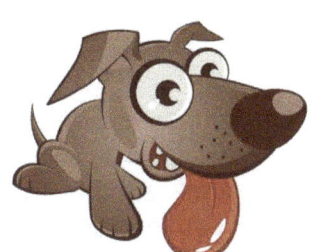

A word of caution: dogs are ardent 'lickers' and it is not always a good idea to put essential oils on your dog's fur as it can be ingested via the licking.

However, you can rub it on your hands before you do any of the 'hands off' work such as scanning the aura, spiralling out pain, tracing pathways etc., and benefit will be felt by your pet. How? Because the therapeutic quality of an essential oil carries a 'vibration' (yes, I was a fan of the Beach Boys, so it could be called a 'good vibration'). That 'vibrational quality' can easily leap the gap between your hand and your dog. So she will receive the therapeutic benefit without risking a reaction to the oil itself.

Be careful with essential oils and if you can, energy test first to ensure it suits your dog and if you are not confident in testing, simply do a patch test to ensure your dog doesn't have a reaction to the oil but _never_ put it undiluted onto her skin.

That said, I have used this following blend for many years and have had no bad reaction.

In a 50ml bottle mix

- Almond oil (or olive or even sunflower, just make sure it is a good quality)
- 10 drops of LAVENDER
- 1 drop TEA TREE – not too much as it can stress the kidney
- 5 drops ROMAN CAMOMILE
- 1 drop LEMONGRASS

You could add a few drops to her shampoo as you will be rinsing it off and you will benefit from a sweet smelling pooch too. In fact, Hippocrates said that the way to health is to have an aromatic bath and scented massage daily ... now I like the sound of that.

So what are the benefits, apart from smelling good?

LAVENDER: if you only buy one oil, buy this one. It's versatile oil that brings the body into general balance and harmony. It's calming and antiseptic. Fantastic for burns and for wound healing. Once the scab has fallen away and there is no risk of infection. Massage a little over the scar, it helps finish off the healing and combined with the massage, helps prevent adhesions. It's a very common oil and is sold everywhere, but buy the best quality organic that you can find; it will have more effective therapeutic properties.

TEA TREE: I am a huge fan of this oil. Anti bacterial, viral, fungus – in fact anti everything. We are now all familiar with the properties of this oil. However, familiarity can breed contempt and always test first as occasionally a dog will find this oil irritating.

ROMAN CAMOMILE: a gentle, warming oil. Safe to use, even on puppies. Soothing and calming. Has been used since ancient times, especially in the Mediterranean and Egypt. Balances the mood and extremely useful for anything to do with 'female' disorders (so this would be one to use after neutering, pregnancy or whelping). Useful for muscle stiffness, inflammation of any kind, indigestion and nausea.

LEMONGRASS: is another one that calms and sedates. This one is particularly useful for total 'overwhelm' that an excessively nervous dog may suffer.

"Look to the perfumes of flowers and of nature, for peace of mind and joy in life" Wang Wei – c. 700AD

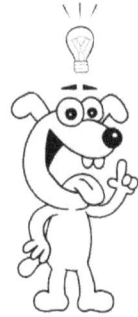

I know I shouldn't really promote – but I have used this particular remedy on myself and my dogs for years and I love it. Nelsons Homeopathic Pharmacy – **Pyrethrum Spray** (takes the mischief out of any insect bites and stings – instantly). About £10 for a small spray that lasts an awfully long time.

www.mobile.nelsonspharmacy.com for online ordering.

Energy Medicine For Your Dog

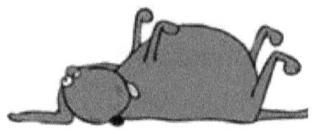

CRYSTALS

I love working with Mother Earth's ancient healers. There are many crystals that can be useful when working with your dog. If you are starting out there are 3 you will enjoy:

- AMETHYST – balance/harmony/back to default
- ROSE QUARTZ – gentle stress reduction/love
- CLEAR QUARTZ – emotional balancer/dispel negativity

Before working with crystals it is essential to cleanse them of any negativity that they may be holding. You want them clean pure and positive.

- Rinse them under running water (cold) – you may like to dip them in salt water, but be careful as some crystals don't like the salt. If in doubt leave the salt out.

- Put them on a wooden board (I use my bread board) and leave them out in the sunshine and moonlight (so an excellent time to do this would be under a full moon). Don't leave them too long in the sunshine, especially if you live in a hot climate, as some crystals fade in the sun. So, say an hour in the sun and all night under moonlight.

- If you have a smudge stick or a good quality incense, pass/fan the smoke over the crystals.

While doing this you can ask the old, stale, tired energy to leave, let all negativity depart and the space be filled with loving, healing, replenishing energy and light.

Remember that all 'working' crystals should be cleansed between techniques by blowing off the tired energy or dipping it in water to wash it off. A full cleaning as outlined above could be done every month, or whenever you fill it is appropriate.

So you now have good, clean and charged crystals and are keen to use them. How do you do that? There are many techniques from simple to complicated. In this booklet here are a couple of techniques that you can't go wrong with.

- Hold your crystal and trace figure 8's over your dog with the crystal.
- Put a crystal under your dog's bed but be careful she can't find it and eat it
- Safely attach one to your dog's collar (make sure she can't loosen and swallow it). You can buy little spiral 'cages' into which you can place a crystal and hang it on the collar.
- Tape a clear quartz to your dog's drinking bowl, which of course, might already have your LOVE & GRATITUDE mat underneath it. Between the two the water will become truly wondrous!

Just for the fun of it, conduct an experiment; put down two identical bowls of water, one with clear quartz + love and gratitude mat and the other with nothing – see which one your dog prefers. If you think your dog might get to the quartz and swallow it simply put it in a jug of water and energise it that way.

Dogs love crystals and often I make a circle of some of the larger ones on my lawn and my dogs always go and sleep or simply sit in the middle of the circle with a soppy look on their faces.

I sometimes bury them under half an inch of earth and leave them for a couple of days to be replenished by Mother Earth herself.

If you are new to crystals just buy simple tumbled versions to start with. I used to get mine from Merton Abbey Mills in Wimbledon www.charliesrockshop.com who do a mail order service. Also the Rock 'n Gem shows around the country are definitely worth a visit.

Normally held at racecourses – www.rockngem.co.uk a great day out and you get good quality crystals at competitive prices.

CHOOSING A VET. Is one of the most important things you will have to do when you get a pet. The very best advice I can give you is to ask around in your area. When I moved I literally went up to every dog owner I saw and asked them who their vet was and were they happy... pretty soon the same name kept coming up and I knew where I was going.

If you are in the London area the vet I would recommend is Mr Richard Bleckman who was awarded 'Vet of the Year' in 2000, he is a very experienced vet that has studied oriental herbal medicines and can therefore offer a fusion of conventional and complementary. Based in Roehampton – take a look at his site for contact details.
www.roehampton-vets.co.uk

Dogs 'bluff' a lot when they meet each other, showing teeth, rising hackles, pawing shoulders but rarely does it go beyond that to a fight. I always look at the owner and if in any doubt (you know what I mean) I walk away and avoid any eye contact. Luckily my little girl is small enough to pick up should I need to.

Ever since Magnus was bitten, I am very nervous when big black dogs come near Mabel, I try not to be but I can't help it; I'm getting better but occasionally there is still a whisper of apprehension. So if that happens, I breathe and tap a magic Triple Warmer Point, telling myself it will be ok and that it is better that I don't fuss or interfere.

So what's that magic TW point? On the top of your hand just below the web between your little and ring finger knuckles, there is a natural indentation. Put your one hand over your heart and with your other hand tap the point on the top of the hand.

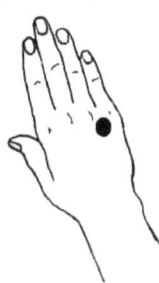
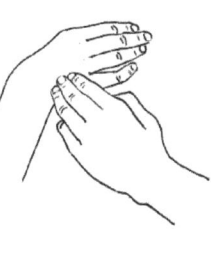

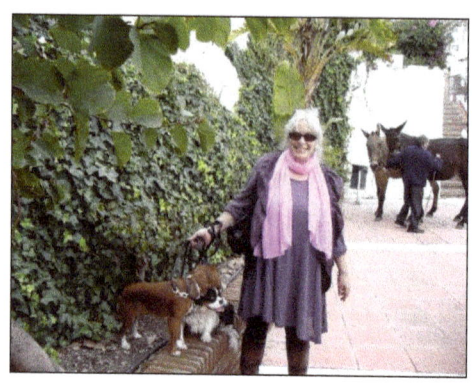

Why did I write this book and who am I?

Well I ask myself the latter a lot! Seriously, I wrote this book because working with energy is such an integral part of my life, it naturally spills over into that of my animals. By osmosis they get energy medicine. It seems to me to be a natural progression from stroking your dog to stroking in a specific way that encourages the flow of energy in her body.

I've always wanted to write a fun little book and I thank my publishers (Caroline and Lynn) for allowing me the freedom to do so now. I hope it will motivate you to experiment with your dog and see which techniques you, and her, enjoy the most. They will then simply weave themselves into your lives, enhancing the already strong bond between the two of you and of course, her health and happiness. Have fun with this, it is nearly all instinctive and a lot you will be doing already.

And me?

Many moons ago I was involved in the heart of London advertising, becoming a successful international board director. However, I realised, after a few ambition fuelled years, that I wanted my life to take a different direction and shocked everyone by giving up the BMW, Armani suits and Gucci briefcase, becoming a student again.

I've trained in massage, sports massage, aromatherapy, Indian head massage, reflexology, trager, nutrition, flower essences, radionics... A true workshop groupie, I proudly filled a wall with qualifications but could not find what I had been seeking; I couldn't even really define it... until, through divine synchronicity, I met Donna Eden in London through a mutual friend. Within no time at all (6 days to be precise), I was in Ashland in Donna's backyard with about four other students, eagerly learning about energy. I remember in those days Donna had two beautiful big dogs – this was more than two decades ago, so no information highway was available and ever the thirsty student, I drank in everything I could on these visits, rushing back to London to experiment on my long suffering clients!

Over the years I crossed the ocean many times learning from Donna and also John Thie [Touch for Health].

I then began to teach Donna's work in many parts of the world. I now divide my time between the Isle of Wight and Andalucía and set up and run the Eden Energy Medicine official training in Europe. It's come a long way since those days in her back yard!

I have published some other books, all available in print or Kindle download from Amazon:

- *Coping with Candida*
- *Stiff Joints*
- *Everyday Energy*

- *MONEY is not a 4 lettered word – connecting to your universal piggy bank*
- *You've got Guts*

And more are in the pipeline.

Animals have always been my passion and shared my life. I suppose my next dream is to sell millions of copies of this book, (or maybe you are a millionaire reading this book and want a project?) and then I could set up an Energy Medicine sanctuary for waifs and strays!

WALKING THE TIGHTROPE

A state of balance is very rarely a truly static state for a human being or any animal. Harmony is like walking a tightrope; we constantly have to move and compensate to maintain our balance. It's a natural dance to be enjoyed and mastered.

I have talked in the book about getting balanced before working on your dog. What do I mean by that? Basically, before working with energy you want to make sure your own in running the right direction, is crossing as it should and is not chaotic or 'scrambled' – it need only take a few seconds, but get into the habit of balancing yourself first, it will make all the difference to the quality and effectiveness of your treatments.

The basic balancing techniques are:

- FOUR 'THUMPS'
- CROSS CRAWL
- TIBETAN MEDITATION POSE
- HOOK UP

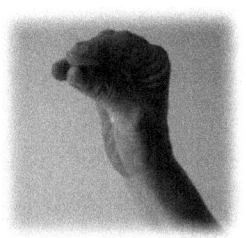

Form your thumb and first two fingers into a triad and firmly massage or tap the points described below.

If you have long nails, simply improvise and use your knuckles. Don't forget to breathe and smile while you tap.

The first 'thump' is K27

The benefits of this simple exercise include:

* 'Flips' energy into forward flow.
* Jump-starts and energises the entire system.
* Balances disruptions caused by travelling, especially through time zones. [A great one to do during a flight and when you step off the plane].
* Brings clarity to thought.
* Improves focus and concentration.
* Brings a flow back into your life.
* Temporarily energises the eyes, useful if you are tired but still have a few more miles to drive.

You will be tapping and therefore stimulating the 27th acupuncture point on each Kidney meridian. These important points act as 'junction boxes' for other meridians.

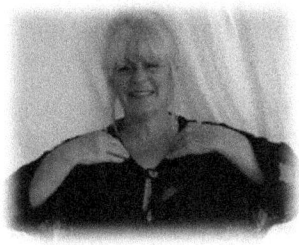

They are located near the 'right angle' where the collar and breast bones meet. You will feel two natural indentations that may be slightly tender when you press them.

Don't worry if you can't find the exact points, you know the approximate area, so tap around and you will get them, as with all energy work, it is about intention and attention.

Breathe, fully moving your rib cage and diaphragm.

Smile and tap for 5 seconds... YES, that's all it takes.

THE TARZAN THUMP!

Benefits of this second thump include:

- Stimulates the Thymus gland.
- Supports the Immune System.
- Helps cope with the body's stress response and negative emotional energies.
- Stimulates overall energy and vitality – primates will thump this gland to increase their strength before mating or fighting.
- Places the body in a temporary state of 'balance'.

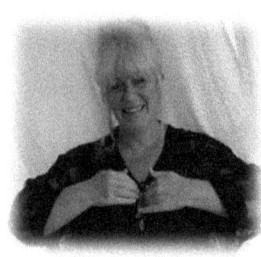

You will be tapping over the Thymus Gland[9] which is located in the middle of your chest – exactly where Tarzan thumps, in fact rather than tapping; you could clench your fists and thump your chest like Tarzan!

Breathe, smile and tap/thump for 5 seconds.

---

[9] The Australian psychiatrist, Dr John Diamond [Your Body Doesn't Lie] www.drjohndiamond.com – made a study of the Thymus gland and suggests we 'waltz' the thymus, i.e. tap lightly to the waltz rhythm... 123 123 123, smile and look at something beautiful while you are tapping to increase the effectiveness of the exercise.

THE MONKEY THUMP

* Benefits of monkey thumping include:
* Boosts Immune System and general energy levels.
* Increases your ability to accept/metabolise changes.
* Balances blood chemistry.
* Aids detoxification of the body.
* Helps metabolise and absorb nutrients.
* Improves absorption of supplements [tap for a few seconds before and after taking them].

You will be massaging/tapping/thumping the 21st acupressure points on each Spleen meridian. These are located on the side of the ribcage, roughly where the bottom line of a bra would sit [see photo]. You will know when you hit on them as they will be tender.

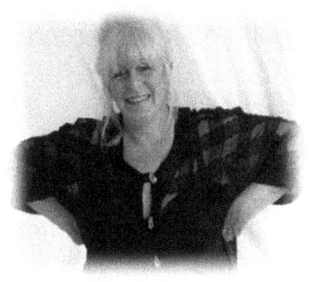

Once located, use your clenched fists to massage, tap or thump firmly the points for a minimum of 5 seconds. Breathe and smile.

You can also work on the Spleen lymphatic points: simply lean back slightly, opening up the ribcage and tap round from Sp21 to underneath each breast in line with the nipples.

CHEEKY THUMP

- Relieves anxiety
- Helps you begin to trust in the mystery of life
- Helps in letting issues pass through, be digested and released
- Balanced Stomach energy encourages you to pay attention to self-care
- Helps achieve a clear thought process.

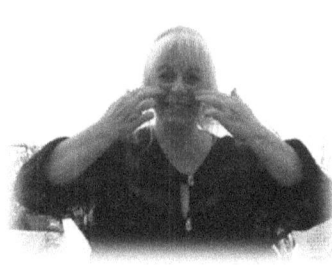

Called the 'Great Bone Hole' they are located slightly below the apex of your cheeks when you smile, in line with your eye and the edge of your nostril.

Again, do for 5 seconds.

THYMUS PRESSURE WITH PRAYER

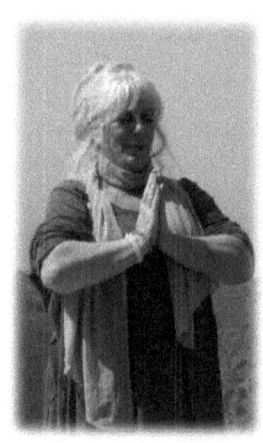

Place your palms together in a prayer position. Forearms parallel with the floor. Thumbs will be over the Thymus gland, push against this point firmly for ten seconds then release. Repeat. This brings you into a temporary state of balance and in the ancient Indian tradition, connects you to your soul.

Say a simple thank you for all your blessings, one of which is your 4-legged friend.

CROSS CRAWL – 20 seconds

The body functions with crossing patterns, curves, roundness and above all, flow. There are very few sharp edges in the human body.

This technique is based on the fact that the left hemisphere of the brain needs to send information to the right side of the body and the right hemisphere to the left side. If either of these 'communication tracts' are not adequately flowing and open then it will be impossible to access the brain's full capacity or the body's full intelligence.

The bottom line is: when our energies are crossed every system in the body and the body's healing abilities is encouraged to optimum efficiency, we are literally healthier. However, when the energies are not crossed, the healing abilities are dramatically reduced.

We are born with the energies running in a parallel pattern, homolaterally[10] down the body but when, as babies, we start to crawl; the crossover pattern and left/right brain integration really begins to take form. This is why children who do not crawl enough can develop learning difficulties. So don't just plonk your baby/grandchild in a bouncer, let it roam wild – the crawling action will enable enhanced brain function.

Back to us as adults: Nature intended that we cross crawl naturally during the course of each day: walking, running, swimming are all natural ways of consolidating that crossing pattern. However, contemporary lifestyles are increasingly sedentary. In addition, fashion footwear can prohibit good posture and, we carry heavy shoulder bags, briefcases or

---

[10] We use the word homolateral to indicate this parallel patterning. II

shopping bags which all inhibit the natural flow of the movement.

Needless to say any stress or trauma in our life can throw the pattern back into homolateral. Our body will give us hints when this happens – for example stop reading right now and see if any 'body part' is crossed – wrists, arms, ankles, legs? This is a message that the body needs/ wants to cross its energies, it yearns to run at full efficiency, it seeks balance to do so.

Body language specialists say crossed arms mean a closed off/ defensive stance, but in reality, from an energetic standpoint, it can also mean that you are trying to cross the energies, albeit unconsciously, so that you can truly understand what is being said to you.

So, to summarise; doing a CROSS CRAWL can improve left and right brain integration and encourage energies to cross.

This in turn can:

Greatly improve the body's natural healing ability.

- Enhance the absorption of vitamin supplementation.
- Relieve fatigue, exhaustion and lack of motivation.
- Bring clarity to your thinking.
- Help your whole system function more efficiently.
- Improve co-ordination.
- Reduce certain learning difficulties.
- Stimulate memory.
- Pump lymphatic and cerebrospinal fluid.
- Help you feel more balanced, motivated and energised.

- Harmonise energies and increase natural self healing abilities.
- Ease depression.
- Support the immune system.
- Support and help make more effective any other treatments you may be receiving from your healthcare practitioner.

It is marching on the spot:
to re-programme the body into a health supporting crossing pattern, without which you will never heal 100%

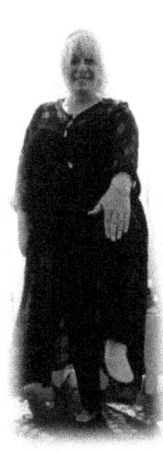

Lift your right arm and right leg together. Then lift your left arm and left leg together. Do you remember the Thunderbird puppets! Repeat a few times/15 seconds or so. This reflects the homolateral, parallel patterning which your brain will recognise and feel comfortable with if your energies are not crossing.

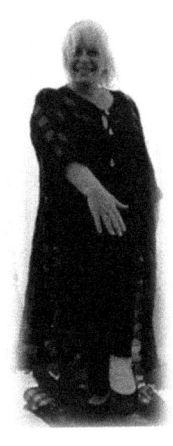

Now lift your right arm and left leg together [see photo on the right above] followed by left arm and right leg. i.e. diagonal/opposites together. Repeat a few times/15 seconds. This represents the crossover pattern and may feel uncomfortable until your energies re-programme themselves into a crossing pattern.

Repeat.

**ALWAYS end on the cross over pattern
and do a few extra 'crosses' to integrate the
reprogramming.**

Unscrambling energy – Tibetan meditation pose

This unscrambles the energies making for clearer communication, clearer thinking, improved left/right brain integration and cheers you up in no time at all, so great for when you are feeling sad, confused or angry. It returns your energy circuits to default, reduces stress, and encourages release of past emotional baggage or trauma.

We tend to naturally sit in this position and it may be familiar to you. It is sometimes considered to be a blocking pose but in reality, if you are over-stimulated, you are naturally trying to unscramble so that you can understand more clearly, so it is the total opposite of being blocked, it is about wanting to be open and understanding.

* Sit [or stand], cross the arms over the chest with hands under the armpits, thumbs out and up.
* Close your eyes, breath and smile.
* Stay in this position until you feel calm.
* Bring your hands into prayer position and take a couple of breaths.
* Put your arms out in front of you, palms facing outwards. Feet are still crossed.
* Cross the wrists and intertwine your fingers, pull them towards you, up and under, so your clasped hands are sitting under your chin. Did you do this when you were a child? I have asked many people

from different countries and most have – as children we instinctively get ourselves into positions that encourage balance.

* Close your eyes, breath and smile. Hold for as long as you want – a minute?

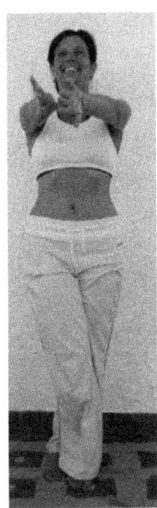
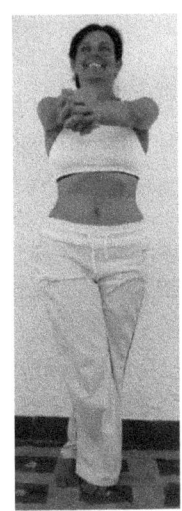
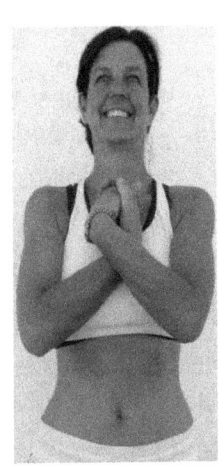

Hook up – a hyperlink to harmony

'Discombobulated' ... I simply love the sound of this word although I have my doubts as to its 'official' existence, but just the sound of it manages to describe how we can all feel occasionally: Uncoordinated in both body and mind; a bit 'off'; a little 'spaced out'; stuck; not fully in the flow of life and unable to cope with the challenges life sets us.

This simple technique is a hyperlink to harmony, equilibrium and balance. It:

- connects [hooks up] two important channels of energies: Governing and Central, which in turn boosts confidence and courage;
- brings clarity of thought and purpose;
- strengthens the auric field, keeping it solid and protective;
- bridges the energies between the head and the body;
- enables you to feel more connected, co-ordinated, grounded and able to cope;
- stimulates the ancient Strangeflow energies.

Place the middle finger of one hand on your forehead between the eyebrows, over the 3rd Eye

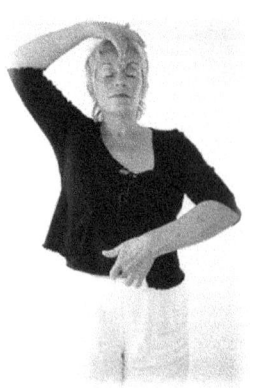

Place the middle finger of the other hand in your navel.

With a slight pull of the skin upward on both points, close your eyes, take a deep breath and relax. [Breathe in through the nose and out through the mouth]

Stay in this position for about twenty seconds [or for however long feels right to you]

By strengthening the Governing Channel that runs up the back, you affect the spine, not only in a physical sense but also in an emotional way – literally giving you the 'backbone' to face and resolve problems and move forward in your life.

By strengthening the Central Channel that runs up the front of the torso you will be less vulnerable to absorbing other peoples' negative energies. An overdose of these can cause exhaustion and even depression.

It is a powerful tool for quickly centring yourself and has immediate neurological consequences. It has been reported to be helpful to a person starting to seizure.

Try it right now and see if you feel less discombobulated!

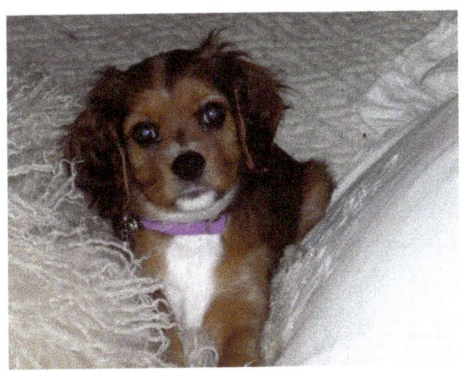

Mabel

I am also adding a little bit more information on how to do a basic energy test, beginners among you might find it useful. Get confident testing the person first and then move on to using them as a surrogate.

> Energy testing enables us to access the body in a language that is easy to understand.
>
> *The body can reveal to us, via the test of applying and resisting pressure on the muscle, if something strengthens or weakens it.*
>
> It is truly that simple.
>
> Of course, nuances have been developed and it has become and 'art and science' but never forget, it is simple, easy, organic, safe and with a little practice – accurate.

Please believe me when I say, that with a little practise, anyone and everyone can do these tests. I am not special; it is neither magic nor trickery. It is a practical bio-feedback tool to help you tune in to your body's needs. Use it with confidence on your children, spouse and friends.

A few preliminaries...

Spend a minute of getting your basic energies balanced (see above).

Make sure they have no injuries or problems that might get in the way of the test. Obviously avoid testing a muscle that is injured or weak for any reason. An accurate result will not be achieved from a shoulder that was dislocated last month!

Neither of you should view this as a competition of strength.

It is also not about 'failure' or 'success' – simply discovering the truth so that we can determine the best way forward for your pet. Especially when it is a surrogate test, they are literally, just a vessel. As one of my teachers once said: *an old garden hose through which the water of information will flow.*

Check their posture is relaxed yet standing straight and nothing is crossed.

Remind them that BREATHING normally is essential throughout – do not hold your breath.

Don't try and second guess the test. Be objective and ready to embrace the truth!

Common sense dictates that the tests will not be accurate if you have taken recreational drugs or alcohol!

Dehydration can affect the test so both of you drink a glass of water beforehand.[11]

Remove any jewellery that may get in the way, watch, bangles etc., IF you think about it, sometimes they do not present a problem. My personal rule of thumb is if I think I about it, I remove it.

Don't energy test right next to a computer or electrical equipment.

Testing is very much of the moment, a present tense. It is not a response of yesterday or tomorrow but very much on now, today. Reflect that in your thinking. Bring all your attention to what you are doing. Very easy with an animal because they live so much in the present moment.

So, put all expectations aside - take a deep breath and get started. Enjoy and relax into it – I was one of Donna's worst students at first because I SO wanted to be the best [let's not even begin to analyse that!] Once I let go, stopped judging myself and relaxed, hey presto – it worked a dream.

---

[11] The test for dehydration is simply to tug at a lock of hair and energy test [ET] if it is weak then dehydration could be an issue

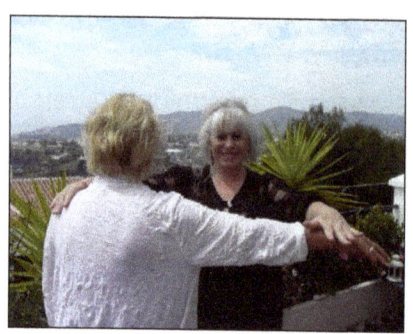

GENERAL INDICATOR MUSCLE
[*Pectoralis Major Clavicular – the smart name for the shoulder muscle which is the one you are isolating and testing*]

Your friend stands up straight, unclenched fists and relaxed, with feet apart. [If necessary, the test can be done sitting].

Left arm [or right] is held out at a right angle to the body and parallel to the floor – you have a range to play with here, from straight out to the side or slightly towards midline, experiment to see what feels right to you.

Check hand is *not* clenched into a fist – fingers should be straight.

Stand in front of your friend, not too close, with your right hand, palm flat and facing downwards and fingers extended – resting on your friend's raised arm, on the forearm just near the wrist joint. [shoulder side of the wrist]. If you test on the other side of the wrist, just the hand will go down not the arm.

The left hand can rest gently on her shoulder to create a full circuit between the two of you.

Demonstrate the range of movement – so that she is confident in what is about to happen. *You are interested in the first couple of inches* of that range, not everyone's arm drops all the way down to their hip. It might be that a 'spongy' response is all that is felt, but that is enough to indicate a weak result.

Tell her to 'HOLD' – wait half a second, while her brain registers the command and then apply pressure for 2 seconds – gently, no jerking movements.

Do not put too much pressure on the arm – the lighter the pressure the better the testing and the less tiring it is for both of you. This becomes particularly relevant when you are doing multiple tests. I often ask students to 'lighten up' even more, they often think it won't work – but it does.

What happened? If it stays in position easily it means that it is testing STRONG.

However, if it is spongy, or falls all the way down then that is a WEAK test.

To get a feel for what is their personal 'yes' and 'no' – try this:

Get them to say the statement 'my name is Minnie Mouse' (without smiling) – energy test – it should be weak, it is a false statement. They could say anything that is false. E.g. my name is Fred, I am standing on the North Pole – anything that is obviously false. Now do the same with a positive statement such as: 'my name is xxyyzzxx' – should be strong.

When you are both balanced and you are confident in the basic energy test, then simply place the surrogate's hand on the dog and test ... it may help to imagine the surrogate's arm as the dog's arm, the surrogate is purely and extension of the dog.

"Kinesiology is based on the fact that the body language never lies. Sometimes we do not understand what the body is trying to tell us, but that does not change the fact that the body is constantly expressing externally what is going on internally."

Sheldon Deal, DC, ND

...and thoughts to the other little feline members of my tribe. I suspect I will be sharing their secrets next!

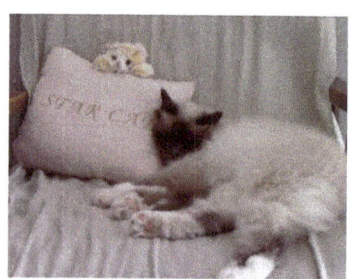
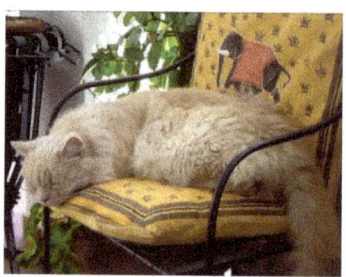

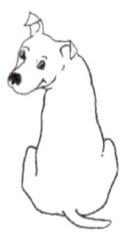

A very special thank you to Anna Maria Paciulli for her canine characters, advice on flower essences and general encouragement over the cosmic airwaves between Italy and Spain!

As always I want to thank Donna Eden without her, I would not be writing this today, it's as simple as that. She and her energy work have been the single biggest influence in my life and I feel a deep gratitude.

And to all the artists at www.Dreamstime.com for some cute illustrations with a high aaahhh factor

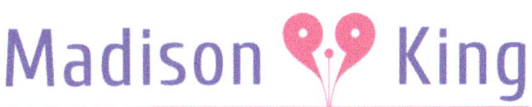

Writer & Teacher of Energy Medicine
madisonking@hotmail.com
FB – Madison's medicine
www.madisonking.com
www.midlifegoddess.ning.com

©July 2014

www.ingramcontent.com/pod-product-compliance
Ingram Content Group UK Ltd.
Pitfield, Milton Keynes, MK11 3LW, UK
UKHW021253180426
11947UKWH00010B/748